FOR REFERENCE

Do Not Take From This Room

Prescription Drugs

Recent Titles in the

CONTEMPORARY WORLD ISSUES
Series

Books in the **Contemporary World Issues** series address vital issues in today's society such as genetic engineering, pollution, and biodiversity. Written by professional writers, scholars, and nonacademic experts, these books are authoritative, clearly written, up to date, and objective. They provide a good starting point for research by high school and college students, scholars, and general readers as well as by legislators, businesspeople, activists, and others.

Each book, carefully organized and easy to use, contains an overview of the subject, a detailed chronology, biographical sketches, facts and data and/or documents and other primary source material, a forum of authoritative perspective essays, annotated lists of print and nonprint resources, and an index.

Readers of books in the Contemporary World Issues series will find the information they need in order to have a better understanding of the social, political, environmental, and economic issues facing the world today.

Prescription Drugs

A REFERENCE HANDBOOK

David E. Newton

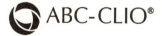

ABC-CLIO®

An Imprint of ABC-CLIO, LLC
Santa Barbara, California • Denver, Colorado

Library of Congress Cataloging-in-Publication Data

Names: Newton, David E., author.
Title: Prescription drugs : a reference handbook / David E. Newton.
Description: Santa Barbara, California : ABC-CLIO, [2022] | Series: Contemporary world issues | Includes bibliographical references and index.
Identifiers: LCCN 2021015458 (print) | LCCN 2021015459 (ebook) | ISBN 9781440877728 (hardcover) | ISBN 9781440877735 (ebook)
Subjects: LCSH: Drugs—Handbooks, manuals, etc.
Classification: LCC RM301.12 .N52 2022 (print) | LCC RM301.12 (ebook) | DDC 615.1—dc23
LC record available at https://lccn.loc.gov/2021015458
LC ebook record available at https://lccn.loc.gov/2021015459

ISBN: 978-1-4408-7772-8 (print)

　　　978-1-4408-7773-5 (ebook)

26 25 24 23 22 　　1 2 3 4 5

This book is also available as an eBook.

ABC-CLIO
An Imprint of ABC-CLIO, LLC

ABC-CLIO, LLC
147 Castilian Drive
Santa Barbara, California 93117
www.abc-clio.com

This book is printed on acid-free paper ∞

Manufactured in the United States of America

Amioderone. Bystolic. Cozar. Finasteride. Lipitor. Lovastatin. Prilosec. Prinivil. Synthroid. Tamsulosin. Xarelto. The names of one or more—often *many* more—prescription drugs would be familiar to nearly all of us. We rely on these drugs to deal with a seemingly endless variety of medical conditions, ranging from pain relief to cure of an infectious disease, to aid in sleeping, to treatment of anxiety or some other mental condition, to preventive purposes such as avoidance of high cholesterol or heart attack.

So it can be a bit surprising to remember that these "miracles" of modern medicine have been available for less than a century. Preventive and curative substances have been around for millennia, of course. And the essential elements of the pharmaceutical industry, such as safe written prescriptions, have existed for more than a hundred years. But the specific chemical compounds we call *prescription drugs* have existed only since 1951, when the U.S. Congress passed the Durham-Humphrey Amendment to the Federal Food, Drug, and Cosmetic Act of 1938. That piece of legislation set in motion the development of a very large, very complex medical, economic, and social system based on the existence and availability of certain compounds that could legitimately be called *prescription drugs*.

That system today consists of very expensive long-term searches for possible prescription drugs, very expensive testing protocols to determine the safety and efficacy of those compounds, very expensive marketing programs to convince health care providers to order and ordinary people to use these drugs, and very expensive challenges to the identification and solution to a variety of social issues arising out of the availability of prescription drugs.

One such challenge in recent decades, for example, has been the rise in illness and death resulting from the illegal, unsafe use of such products, for purposes for which they were not intended. For much of the 2010s, the so-called *opioid epidemic* was the most serious health care issue in the United States and other parts of the world. The conclusion of that period saw a very different—but also very troublesome—new problem: the rising cost of prescription drugs. By 2020, vast numbers of Americans had begun to realize that (1) they had become dependent on the availability of prescription drugs for all manner of medical conditions, ranging from annoying skin rashes to potentially fatal organ failure, and (2) they too often could not afford the prescription drugs they had come to rely on for a safe, healthy, happy life. The nation had fallen into an economic cataclysm of skyrocketing drug prices.

These and other prescription drug issues affect Americans of every sex, gender, age, race, ethnicity, and other characteristic. We begin with a review of the history and background of prescription drugs: when and where they were discovered, how the field of pharmacology developed, what have been the basic factors that led to each of the problems we face today. These topics are the focus of Chapter One.

Chapter Two turns more specifically to the status of the prescription drug industry today. What are the major challenges for that industry and the general public at large? What solutions to those problems have been proposed, tried, and found to succeed or fail?

Chapter Three is a section of special interest to many readers. It is a collection of essays on special issues in the field of prescription drugs of technical or personal interest to the average person. The remaining chapters of the book are designed to assist those readers who want to learn more about the topic of prescription drugs and/or to continue their own research on

the topic. They include information on important individuals and organizations in the field (Chapter Four), current data
about and documents relating to the subject (Chapter Five),
an annotated bibliography of more than a hundred valuable
resources on prescription drugs (Chapter Six), a chronology
of important events in the field of prescription drugs (Chapter
Seven), and a glossary of useful terms in the field.

Prescription Drugs

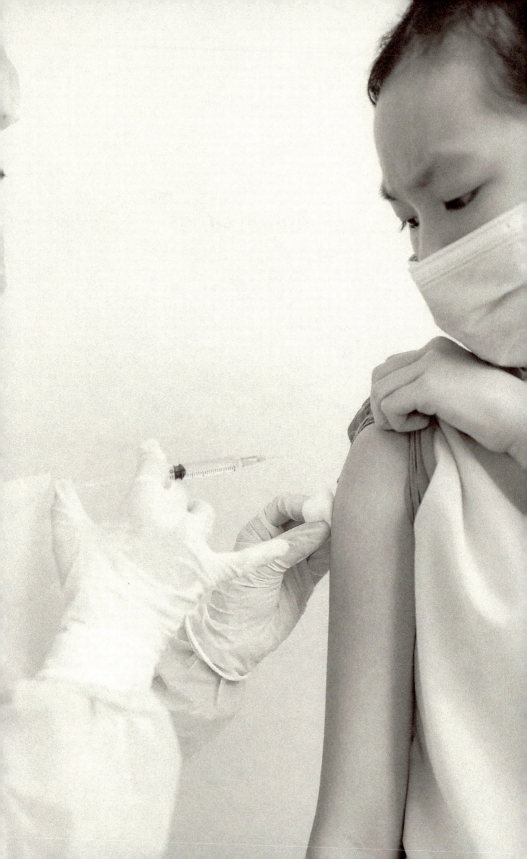

In December 2019, public health officials in Wuhan, China, reported the appearance of a new type of pneumonia among forty-one patients in the city. Within a month, Chinese researchers identified the causative agent to be a previously unknown form of a coronavirus, a type of virus that causes several types of respiratory disorders, ranging from simple flu-like conditions to more serious disorders such as Middle East respiratory syndrome (MERS) and severe acute respiratory syndrome (SARS). The new virus was later named coronavirus-19 (indicating that it is the nineteenth form of coronavirus discovered). The disease it causes was labeled COVID-19.

Some political leaders worldwide viewed the new disease as "just one more kind of flu" that would soon "go away" on its own. But events proved that hope to be unfounded. The disease soon spread to Thailand, South Korea, Iran, Italy, Philippines, Spain, and the United States. Public health experts also discovered that the death rate from the disease was nearly fifty times as great as that from the common flu, with which it was sometimes being compared (Secon 2020). Health officials and government leaders soon began to realize that aggressive action was necessary to bring the disease under control. They recommended or mandated well-known pandemic health measures, such as social distancing, the wearing of masks, and increased attention to personal hygiene.

A doctor administers the COVID-19 vaccine to a woman to produce immunity against the coronavirus disease. (Satjawat Boontanataweepol/ Dreamstime.com)

The results of these new measures were mixed. In some countries, the rate of infection decreased significantly, although the disease continued to spring up in new locations and increased in many others. It was not long before those in authority realized—as had many medical experts—that the disease would be brought under control only with the development of new drugs and/or vaccines. But that remedy had its own problems. The discovery, manufacture, and approval of a new drug takes, on average, about ten years. The likelihood of a candidate drug's reaching the marketplace is only 12 percent, and the cost of even getting to the drug approval phase averages about $2.6 billion ("Biopharmaceutical Research & Development" 2015). Under those conditions, the chance of having a new COVID-19 drug available in the near future (a few months or even a year or two) was slim. In order to speed up this process, the U.S. government, and other governments around the world, poured grant money in the drug discovery and development process, hoping to speed up the process required to get the new vaccine or drug. Why did this process take so long?

For readers of this book, this story might raise many questions about drugs. What, after all, is a "drug"? Are all drugs "prescription drugs"? Why or why not? Is a vaccine a drug? Are there other kinds of drugs besides prescription drugs? If so, what are they? How are they different from prescription drugs (if at all)? Why is it so expensive to make a new drug? Why does it take so long to produce one? Why and how is the federal government involved in this process? What does it mean to say that a drug is "approved"? How important is the approval process?

Drug Basics

Many definitions have been suggested for the term *drug*. One of the best authorities in this regard is the U.S. Food and Drug Administration (FDA). The FDA offers four different, but complementary, definitions for the term. The one most commonly found, and the one used for this book, is as follows:

A substance intended for use in the diagnosis, cure, mitigation, treatment, or prevention of disease. (Drugs@FDA Glossary of Terms 2017)

Another definition used by the FDA is as follows:

A substance recognized by an official *pharmacopoeia* or *formulary*.

A pharmacopoeia is an official publication that lists all drugs currently in use, their physical, chemical, and biological properties; their effects on the human body; and their directions for use. The United States Pharmacopoeia (USP) is an organization made up of experts in the field of drugs that publishes a book by that name. USP also has several other functions, such as testing the quality, strength, purity, safety, and other properties of drugs ("What Is the U.S. Pharmacopeia?" 2015). A drug formulary is similar to a pharmacopoeia in that it lists and describes drugs, but it lists only prescribed drugs. The term may also refer to the prescribed drugs that are covered by some health plan, for example, Medicare.

Drug Sources

Some drugs consist of natural products; others are made synthetically. A third category of drugs is called *semi-synthetic*, because they are made by modifying natural products to make them more effective, safer, less expensive, or different in some other way from the original natural product. Probably the best example of a natural drug is aspirin. Historians believe that aspirin was first used as a drug in about 1934 BCE. It was extracted from the bark of the willow tree and originally called *salicin*. (In modern terminology, the willow tree belongs to the genus *Salix*.) Salicin was used to reduce pain and fever in a patient. Chemists later discovered that the active chemical in salicin is a compound called *salicylic acid*. They found a way of improving the effectiveness of salicin by converting salicylic acid to *sodium salicylate*, the active ingredient in modern aspirin. Therefore, aspirin can also be thought of as a semi-synthetic drug (Desborough and Keeling 2017).

Natural drugs are still widely used today. In fact, many people believe that natural products should be used whenever possible rather than synthetic products. Among the most popular natural drugs are herbs such as Taxol, extracted from the bark of the Pacific yew tree and used to treat cancer; ginger (*Zingiber officinale*), recommended for the treatment of vomiting and nausea, menstrual pain, and a host of other disorders; and aloe vera, used to reduce pain, inflammation, and swelling (Khan and Abourashed 2013).

Some of the most problematic drugs known, the so-called *drugs of abuse*, are most commonly natural drugs or semi-synthetic products made from those materials. They include drugs such as cocaine, opium and its derivatives, psilocybin, cannabis, tobacco, and khat. Drugs in this category play an outsized role in the history of prescription drugs, as will be seen later in this book.

The vast majority of drugs available in the world today are synthetic products, compounds made artificially in a chemistry laboratory. For example, of the ten drugs most commonly prescribed in the United States in 2020, nine were synthetic compounds. Only one, levothyroxine, did not fall into that category. It is a semi-synthetic product ("ClinCalc DrugStats Database" 2021).

Drug Types

All drugs used in the United States must be approved by the FDA. Those drugs are divided into two main categories: prescription drugs and over-the-counter drugs. The term *prescription drug* is often abbreviated as Rx. The common abbreviation for *over-the-counter* is OTC. Prescription drugs can be obtained by a consumer only with a written order from a licensed health care practitioner, such as a physician, physician's assistant, nurse, dentist, veterinarian, or pharmacist. OTC drugs can be purchased without a prescription, simply by picking them up at a drug store or other distributor. Among the most common OTC drugs, by category, are acid reducers, hand sanitizers, nonsteroidal anti-inflammatory drugs (NSAIDs), cold medications, muscle relaxants, cough suppressants, allergy medications, and drugs for upset stomach.

Several differences exist between prescription and OTC drugs. Individual consumers can decide which OTC drugs they want to buy and how to use them. By contrast, prescription drugs are designated for one specific person, to be used in a precise way. Also, the approval process for prescription drugs involves a higher standard of safety than that for OTC drugs. Prescription drugs also tend to be stronger than OTC drugs. OTC drugs are available in a wide variety of stores, including about 750,000 retail outlets in the United States, versus about 55,000 pharmacies at which prescription drugs can be obtained. The approval process for the two types of drugs is different. A prescription drug must pass through a process called New Drug Application (NDA; described later), while an OTC drug is regulated by a document called a *monograph*. A monograph lists all of the relevant conditions needed for an approved OTC drug, such as acceptable ingredients, dosages, formulations, and labeling. Finally, OTC drugs are required to have a label known as the *drug facts* label. That label provides all the information a consumer needs to make an intelligent choice of OTC drugs. It contains a list of active ingredients and a list of inactive ingredients, drug uses, warnings about its uses, and directions for use. Most of this information is omitted from a prescription drug label because the FDA's approval process and health care specialist's knowledge of the drug have confirmed the information. (For more on drug facts, see "OTC Drug Facts Label" 2015.)

Drugs can also be classified according to the purpose for which they are used. Some common categories are as follows:

- analgesics: relief of pain
- antacids: reduction of stomach acid and accompanying symptoms

- antianxiety drugs: reduction of anxiety attacks
- antiarrhythmics: treatment of irregular heartbeat
- antibacterials: treatment of infection
- antidepressants: mood lifters
- antiemetics: treatment of nausea and vomiting
- anti-inflammatories: reduction of inflammation
- antipyretics: reduction of fever
- cough suppressants: treatment of throat irritation and/or coughing
- diuretics: increase the flow of urine
- laxatives: increase the frequency and comfort of bowel movements
- tranquilizers: produce a calming or relaxing effect

For a detailed listing of drug types and examples, see "Category Names, Results, and Descriptions" (2020). This list includes both prescription and OTC drugs.

A variety of resources are available for finding and learning about any specific prescription drug. Probably the most readily available and complete of those resources is the FDA's *Approved Drug Products with Therapeutic Equivalence Evaluations*, commonly known as the Orange Book. That publication is available in an interactive format on the Internet, at https://www.fda.gov/drugs/drug-approvals-and-databases/approved-drug-products-therapeutic-equivalence-evaluations-orange-book. The book is updated on an annual basis.

The field of drugs in general is a very large and complex one. The FDA has estimated that more than 20,000 prescription drugs have been approved in the United States for marketing and use. To make the topic easier to understand and study, other systems are also available for classifying drugs. One of the most important of those categories includes *vaccines*. A vaccine is a substance that simulates the body's immune system so as to protect the body from future infections. Most people in developed countries now routinely have vaccinations for several diseases that can otherwise be harmful and event fatal, including diphtheria, measles, mumps, polio, rubella, smallpox, tuberculosis, and varicella. For a list of vaccines commonly in use in the United States, see "List of Vaccines Used in the United States" (2018).

The search for a tool to deal with COVID-19, described previously, focused on both a drug—a substance to *cure* the disease—and a vaccine—a substance to *prevent* a person's catching the disease in the first place. A vigorous debate over the use of vaccines has been going on in the United States and most other parts of the world for many years. For more background on that debate, see Davidson (2019).

Another category of drugs of considerable significance today involves products with the potential for dependence, addiction, and other forms of abuse. Perhaps best known among these drugs are alcohol, cocaine, heroin, LSD, cannabis, and prescription opioids. These drugs are of special interest not only because of their profound health effects on individuals and the issues they create for society at large but also because of their critical role in the history of prescription drugs (as discussed later). In the United States and other countries, systems have been developed to control the manufacture, release, and use of these drugs of abuse. In this country, control of that system resides in the U.S. Drug Enforcement Administration (DEA) and is based on a system created by the Controlled Substances Act of 1970. That system consists of five "Schedules" based in general on two factors: the drug's potential for beneficial use in medicine and its potential for abuse by a user. More detail on the specific criteria for the Schedules can be found at "The Controlled Substances Act" (n.d.). Table 1.1 shows a summary of the five Schedules that make up this system, along with some of the best known members of each Schedule.

Table 1.1 Drug Schedules

Schedule	Criteria	Examples
I	No currently accepted medical use High potential for abuse	Heroin Hallucinogens (e.g., LSD) Marijuana (cannabis) MDMA (Ecstasy) Peyote
II	Some currently accepted medical use(s) High potential for abuse, including severe psychological or physical dependence	Cocaine Morphine Opium Methadone Oxycodone Hydrocodone Fentanyl Amphetamine Methylphenidate
III	Some currently accepted medical use(s) Moderate to low potential for abuse	Anabolic steroids Ketamine Testosterone Low-dose codeine
IV	Generally accepted medical use(s) Low potential for abuse	Ambiem Ativan Librium Lunesta Diazepam Tramadol Xanax
V	Generally accepted medical use(s) Lowest potential for abuse May contain limited amounts of narcotics	Antidiarrheals Antitussives Analgesics

Many of the compounds found in the drug Schedules list are *narcotics*. A narcotic is formally defined as any compound that dulls the senses, relieves pain, and/or produces other physical or mental effects on a person. Recently, the DEA adopted a new definition of the term, referring to a specific class of compounds: opium, opium derivatives, and semi-synthetic compounds of opium. Among the specific drugs covered by this term are opium itself, codeine, morphine, fentanyl, methadone, ocycodone, hydrocodone, hydromorphone, and meperidine ("Narcotics [Opioids]" n.d.).

Drug Nomenclature

Most prescription drugs have three kinds of names: chemical names; generic or nonproprietary names; and trade, or brand, names. Many people are familiar with the drug known as Lipitor, prescribed to treat cholesterol imbalance. At one time, Lipitor was the most widely prescribed drug in the United States. Lipitor is the trade, or brand, name for a compound known as atorvastatin. Atorvastatin is the generic name for the drug, which is also marketed under more than one hundred trade names, of which Lipitor is only the most famous. (See, for example, https://www.medindia.net/drugs/trade-names/atorvastatin.htm for a list of these names.) Most brand names are trademarked by the companies that make them, so that one often sees "Lipitor" written as "Lipitor®," indicating that the manufacturer of that drug has claimed individual control over that name.

Generic names are selected by drug manufacturers to describe specific chemical compounds they have developed. Thus, one can come across many different names for the compound atorvastatin. But no matter the specific trade name used, the basic chemical composition of these drugs is essentially the same. (For more on the naming of generic drugs, see https://www.pfizer.com/news/hot-topics/ever_wonder_how_drugs_are_named_read_on.)

Table 1.2 lists the generic and brand names of some common prescription drugs.

In view of this discussion, one might ask why a drug manufacturer does not simply use the exact chemical name for the drug that they have developed. The answer is simple: those chemical names are almost always so complex that they are difficult to use in everyday life. Although they must be used in scientific literature in discussing a particular drug, for everyday conversation, its essential to have a shorter "nickname" for the drug, the generic name. As an example of this fact, have a look at the chemical name of atorvastatin: (3R,5R)-7-[2-(4-fluorophenyl)-3-phenyl-4-(phenylcarbamoyl)-5-propan-2-ylpyrrol-1-yl]-3,5-dihydroxyheptanoic acid.

Table 1.2 Some Common Generic and Brand Names

Generic Name	Brand Name*
Acetaminophen	Tylenol
Adalimumab	Humira
Albuterol	AccuNeb, Proair, Proventil, Ventolin
Alprazolam	Xanax
Atorvastatin	Lipitor
Azithromycin	Zithromax
Diazepam	Valium
Esomeprazole	Nexium
Finasteride	Proscar, Propecia
Fluoxetine	Prozac
Fluticasone	Flonase
Gabapentin	Neurontin
Ibuprofen	Advil, Motrin
Levothyroxine	Synthroid
Lisinopril	Zestril, Prinzide
Lovastatin	Mevacor
Metformin	Glucophage
Methylphenidate	Concerta
Naloxone	Narcan, Evzio
Omeprazole	Prilosec
Phenytoin	Dilantin
Prednisone	Delatsone
Pregabalin	Lyrica
Ranitidine	Zant
Rivaroxaban	Xarelto
Sertraline	Zoloft
Simvastatin	Zocor
Tamsulosin	Flomax
Zolpidem	Ambien

*More than one brand name may be available.

The Drug Approval Process

The process by which a new drug becomes available to the marketplace has changed dramatically over the centuries. In the earliest periods of human history, the identification of a possible therapeutic product was almost certainly trial and error. In looking for a way to cure headaches, for example, a priest, shaman, or other "wise man (or woman)" probably simply tried one natural product after another before finding something that worked (hopefully, not killing many individuals in the process). Observing the effect of plants and minerals on humans and other animals may also have led to some drug products.

Preclinical Testing

Over time, this process has become far more sophisticated, resulting in a process today that is highly complex, lengthy, and very carefully monitored by governmental agencies. The first step in that process takes place within a chemistry laboratory or, in many cases, several chemistry laboratories working on the same or similar medical problems. The goal of this research is to identify a *target* for the new drug, a biochemical entity that is known or thought to be associated with some specific medical problem. Such structures are also known as *druggable targets*. For example, researchers have found certain genes, proteins, or other structures that, when they appear in an organism, may cause the development of a cancer. This first step in the drug development process includes a review of drug target databases, websites that list all known targets for certain types of disease or disorder. A program known as PharmMapper, for example, lists more than 53,000 chemical structures known to be associated with some type of biological activity (Ajami and Buvailo 2017).

The next step in the drug development process involves finding small molecules that will combine with and activate the targeted site. Again, in many cases, this information may already be available from a database, although a researcher usually has to sift through many possible molecules in order to determine these so-called fits. One might discover a dozen or more fits for any given target entity, so the next step is to find out which of those fits is the best available, meaning that it most efficiently activates the target without causing some sort of damage to it. That "best available fit" is called the *lead compound*; it is the fit a researcher thinks most likely to lead to a new drug (Hughes, et al. 2011). In many cases, there are more than one lead compounds, requiring further research to determine the one most likely to be a drug. That compound is called the *candidate* compound (Hefti 2008).

The next stage in the development process is *preclinical testing*, that is, a series of tests to be completed before the drug is tested in humans. Two types of tests are conducted at this stage: *in vitro* and *in vivo*. The term *in vitro* means "in glass," and it refers to tests that can be conducted on the candidate molecule in a test tube, flask, or other piece of laboratory hardware. The term *in vivo* means "in living object" and involves tests on experimental animals, such as mice and rats. The main purpose of these tests is to determine the safety of a candidate compound, although efficacy of the compound is also important.

Clinical Testing

The success rate for a candidate drug at the end of the preclinical process was about 14 percent during the period 2006 to 2010. That rate had been substantially different in the preceding years, reaching a high of 44 percent from 1996 to 2000 to its lowest point in the period 2006 to 2010 (Takebe, Imai, and Ono 2018). Those data mean that, for the latest dates available, about one out of seven chemical compounds had performed well enough in the first stages of drug development to go on to clinical trials, the next stage in that process.

For successful drug candidates, the next stage of development involves a series of three (sometimes four) clinical tests. Clinical testing for prescription drugs consists of a series of tests to determine whether a candidate compound is (1) safe and (2) effective for use in humans. Such tests are conducted with human volunteers who agree to take part in a trial for a variety of reasons. Some people do so just because they want to contribute to the advance of knowledge about medical conditions. Others sign up in an effort to deal with their own medical condition, which may not have been helped by any other form of treatment.

The key element in finding volunteers for clinical trials is *informed consent*. This phrase means that a prospective volunteer clearly understands all the risks and benefits that may result from the experiment. The candidate drug may have no effect at all on a human, contribute to a cure for a disease, or cause grievous harm (even death) to the volunteer. Most colleges, universities, and other research institutions have standing committees to make sure that all testing done by researchers with whom they are affiliated guarantees informed consent as part of the experimental design. A set of regulations for obtaining informed consent by one major research company can be found at "Chapter XIII—Requirements for Informed Consent" (n.d.).

Another important challenge in selecting volunteers for clinical testing is intentional or unintentional bias in selecting volunteers. For example, the fraction of women, African American, Hispanic, Asian, or other class of volunteers in any one trial for a new drug might be less, often much less, than that in the general population. As a result, the information gained from a clinical test might be appropriate and valid for white males, who make up the largest fraction of the volunteer population, but not necessarily for women or minorities. If all humans of every description always respond to chemical treatments in the same way, this bias would not be relevant. But such is not the case. African American women, for example, might respond in significantly different ways to a drug than do white men. This problem is one that has troubled researchers for many years, a concern for which a variety of solutions have been suggested (Fisher and Kalbaugh 2011).

As Table 1.3 shows, clinical testing usually consists of four stages, although a fifth stage (Phase 0) may also be used. The focus of the earliest stages of testing, Phase I, is the safety of the candidate drug. If the compound causes significant health issues for volunteers, then there is no chance of its ever being approved by the FDA. Testing at this stage usually involves a handful of volunteers, generally fewer than a hundred people,

Table 1.3 Stages of Clinical Testing of Candidate Drugs

Phase	Number of Volunteers	Primary Goal	Dose	Success Rate*
0	Fewer than 10	Biological properties of the drug	Not relevant	Not relevant
I	Fewer than 100	Safety of drug	Less than therapeutic, but increased during testing	75%
II	100–300	Side effects and efficacy	Therapeutic	50%
III	300–3,000	Efficacy and safety in patients with condition	Therapeutic	59%
IV	Unlimited	Post-marketing surveillance	Therapeutic	88%

*Data from Takebe, Imai, and Ono 2018.
Therapeutic dose = dose expected to be used if drug is approved.

preferably in a ratio of sex, race, ethnic group, and other characteristics that is typical of the general population. Phase I testing may take anywhere from about a week to many months.

Early in Phase I of the testing cycle, a manufacturer is required to submit to the FDA a form known as an Investigational New Drug (IND) application. That application alerts the FDA to the manufacturer's intent and outlines any previous research conducted on the drug. The IND application releases the manufacturer from most of the FDA regulations that a researcher would otherwise have to observe ("Investigational New Drug Application" 2020).

Phase II shifts focus somewhat from safety concerns to measurements of efficacy. That is, does the candidate compound actually have any effect on the disease for which it is designed? On average, 100 to 300 volunteers with the specific disease being studied are selected for the study. A variety of experimental designs can be used for these studies. One type might be a *randomized controlled trial,* in which some volunteers are given the experimental drug, while others are given either a placebo, a compound that has no therapeutic effect, or an existing drug used to treat the condition being studied. About a third of the drugs that start Phase I get through to Phase II. Phase II tends to last about two years.

Phase III represents an "all-out" attack on a disease with the candidate drug. A much larger volunteer population is used, up to about 3,000 people, with an examination of all possible safety, efficacy, and side effects being studied. Tests are designed to match real-life situations as closely as possible. Those tests are likely to last anywhere from one to about four years. Roughly, one in five drugs that enter Phase I of clinical testing successful pass through to Phase III.

FDA Approval

The successful completion of Phase III testing permits a manufacturer to submit the new drug to the FDA for approval. That application form, called a New Drug Application (NDA), provides all the information a manufacturer has collected about a drug, including chemical studies, experimental animal research, and clinical trial information. The FDA review committee then has up to six months to decide whether or not to approve the new drug for marketing and consumer use ("New Drug Application [NDA]" 2019).

One of the key components of the FDA review is its assessment of the proposed drug label. To the average person, the term *label* probably means the label attached to the bottle containing a drug. That is one definition of the term. More generally, the term refers to all items that contain information about the drug, including the label on a box or other container in which the drug is made available, and, most important, the printed insert included within the container. That insert contains all essential information about the drug needed by a prescriber or a user of the drug. It lists such information as warnings about use of the drug, indications and usages, dosage and administration, forms and strengths available, contraindications, warnings and precautions, possible adverse reactions, drug interactions, and use in specific populations. A completed drug label can easily run four, five, or more pages (Lal and Kremzner 2017); for a suggested drug label template, see "Prescription Drug Labeling Resources" (2020).

Phase IV of the drug development process is also referred to as *post-marketing surveillance* (PMS). Although a drug is thoroughly tested in Phases I through III of the clinical testing stage of the procedure, some questions always remain once the drug is available in the marketplace. Perhaps most important of these questions is what side effects or other *adverse events* may occur as the result of long-term use of the drug. Preapproval tests run no more than a few years, but many drugs in real life are used by patients for dozens of years. In such cases, issues may arise that were not foreseen during the original approval process, and the FDA may decide to take action on limiting or recalling the drug in question. Phase IV testing also differs from other stages of the process because of the number of subjects involved, often hundreds of thousands or millions of patients compared to just a few thousands during clinical trials (Suvarna 2010).

In its revised regulatory scheme for drug development in 2006, the FDA announced a new level of the approval process, designated as Phase 0. A relatively small number of drugs pass through this stage. It is conducted to see if the basic properties needed by a new drug are met by the candidate compound. Tests are conducted at very low doses, usually about 1 percent that of a therapeutic dose, on no more than ten volunteers for a period of about a week. Even this brief test will show if a candidate compound is safe enough to use in the remaining stages of the drug development process (Kummar, et al. 2008).

Unapproved Drugs

The preceding discussion might lead one to think that prescription drugs used in the United States are always completely safe and effective. That belief is probably largely true, but it ignores the fact that a considerable number of drugs currently in use have not been formally approved by the FDA. The main reason for this situation is that the FDA itself has existed only since 1906 and the requirement that drugs be safe has been around only since 1938. The restriction that they must be both safe *and* effective, in turn, has existed only since 1962. Given that history, the fact remains that many drugs that had been in use in the United States for a century or more, or even for a much shorter time, have never gone through the approval process. These drugs are, in general, *grandfathered in*, that is, allowed to remain in circulation because they *probably* are safe and effective.

The FDA continuously attempts to reduce the number of these unapproved drugs. In 2011, for example, it issued a document ("Guidance for FDA Staff and Industry" 2011) explaining how manufacturers could proceed to have their current unapproved drugs screened and approved by the FDA. As of late 2020, the U.S. National Library of Medicine listed 1,207 drugs in use that had not yet been approved by the FDA ("Unapproved Drugs" 2020); also see "Guidance for FDA Staff and Industry" (2011).

A class of drugs also considered to be "unapproved" are so-called *off-label drugs*, or drugs that have *off-label uses*. An off-label use is some application of a compound in circumstances for which it was not originally intended and for which it was not approved by the FDA. Perhaps the most common off-label use in the United States involves the drug gabapentin. Gabapentin was approved by the FDA in 2011 for the treatment of epilepsy and some forms of neuropathy (nerve pain). Rather quickly, physicians began to realize that the drug could also be used for a variety of other medical conditions not mentioned in the original FDA approval document. These conditions include attention deficit disorders, bipolar disease, restless leg syndrome, and many forms of pain therapy. According to some studies, these off-label uses of gabapentin may account for more than 90 percent of all prescriptions written for the drug (Peckham, et al. 2018). This practice is not prohibited by law, and physicians may prescribe a drug for off-label uses without penalty. For other examples of off-label use, see "Off-Label Drug Prescribing: What Does It Mean for You?" (2015).

Orphan Drugs

A special category of FDA-approved drugs includes the so-called *orphan drugs*. An orphan drug is a product developed and used for the treatment of rare diseases (or *orphan diseases*), which affects a small number of patients. "Small," according to the FDA, means a medical condition that affects fewer than 200,000 people in the United States. Historically, the cost of developing drugs for this relatively small number of patients was greater than manufacturers were willing to spend, based on the profit they could expect to make. For example, only ten drugs meeting the criteria of orphan drugs were approved in the United States between 1973 and 1983 ("Developing Products for Rare Diseases & Conditions" 2018).

In 1983, the U.S. Congress passed the Orphan Drug Act, providing incentives to drug manufacturers to invent, develop, and market such drugs. Among those incentives were grants to drug manufacturers to cover some of the cost of drug development, waivers of or reductions in fees normally charged during the drug development process, a substantial tax credit to companies for expenses incurred in the development of an orphan drug, and an extension in the period of time over which a company had exclusive rights to the ownership, production, and sale of the drug (Seoane-Vazquez, et al. 2008).

As of 2018, a total of 503 drugs had been approved by the FDA by way of the orphan drugs program. A current complete list of orphan drugs is available on the FDA's website, at https://rarediseases.info.nih.gov/diseases/fda-orphan-drugs. The program continues to be the subject of controversy and debate, however, as to its effectiveness in reaching the 1983 Act's original goals. For example, also as of 2018, no therapeutic options had been developed for 95 percent of rare diseases. Also, an implied goal of the Act, namely, to keep orphan drug prices under control, appears to have been less than successful. By 2017, the average price of an orphan drug in the United States had reached twenty-five times the price of non-orphan products. That average price in 2017 was $186,758 for a one-year treatment. The annual cost for the ten most expensive orphan drugs in the world ranged from a high of $1,210,000 (Glybera from uniQure) to a low of $450,540 (Folotyn from Spectrum Pharmaceuticals) (Carroll 2017). A good general summary of the status of orphan drugs is available at "The Rise of Orphan Drugs" (2019).

Prescription Drugs in History

When was the first prescription written? There is almost certainly no definitive answer to that question. Throughout all of human history, humans appear to have had a certain class of individuals who have had the knowledge and skills needed for the care of human health. These healers, shamans, witch doctors, sorcerers, priests—by whatever name they were called—often wrote down "recipes" for curing disease and treating injuries. The current abbreviation for *prescription*, Rx, comes from the Latin word for *recipe, recipere,* which means "to take." Some authorities date the earliest written prescriptions to about 3000 BCE, based on a Sumerian clay table containing instructions for preparing fifteen concoctions for the treatment of disease (Teall 2014); dates for most early events are often the subject of considerable debate. Some authorities date the Sumerian tablets in question to closer to 2100 BCE. One of the prescriptions calls for the use of the bark of an apple tree for cleansing a wound, corresponding to a considerable degree the procedures followed today.

Over time, these sets of prescribing instructions became larger, more specific, and more extensive. For example, the first materia medica (collection of drugs and prescriptions) is sometimes credited to the work of Chinese emperor Shen Nung, in about 2000 BCE. And perhaps the most famous of all early works of this type can be found in the Ebers papyrus from about 1500 BCE in ancient Egypt. That work contains more than 900 prescriptions that make use of more than 700 drugs (Wagner 2019). In terms of long-term influence, perhaps the most important figure in this field is the Roman herbalist Pedanius Dioscorides, who worked primarily from about 50 to 70 CE. Dioscorides wrote a five-volume work on the use of herbs and minerals for the treatment of disease. He included more than 600 substances for use with more than a thousand medical problems. Dioscorides's book was the most influential book in herbalism for more than 1,500 years (Osborn 2018).

The History of Pharmaceutics

Well into the first millennium of the current era (at least 1000 CE), little difference existed between the fields of medicine and pharmacy. Today, we use the term *medicine* to describe the study and treatment of physical and mental problems, reserving *pharmacy* for the study and utilization of drugs for medical use. During early periods, a shaman, healer, or physician would be expected to carry out both activities, learning about herbs and minerals effective for the treatment of disease and injury and then putting that knowledge to work in the treatment of such conditions. For a superb illustrated history of pharmacy, see the collection of paintings at Hanneman (2014).

The first important break between these great traditions came sometime between 1231 and 1240, when the German emperor Frederick II issued what some historians have called "the Magna Carta of the profession of pharmacy." That edict established a clear distinction between the fields of medicine and pharmacy through a set of three innovations. First, the edict specifically noted that the practices of the two sciences required different kinds of knowledge and skills and, therefore, training and practice of the two should be distinct from each other. The second feature of the edict was the recognition that pharmaceutical activities had real and direct influence on the general public and that, therefore, they should be regulated by some governmental agency. Third, to further ensure the quality of drugs produced and distributed by pharmacists, members of that profession should be required to take an oath that the materials they produced were safe and effective (Kremers, Urdang, and Sonnedecker 1976/1986).

It was at this point that the two fields of medicine and pharmacy began to grow apart from each other, with separate professional organizations and training facilities being developed for each of the two subjects. For example, the world's first pharmacy was founded in Florence in 1221, just prior to Frederick's edict. It is said that the Dominican monks who founded the business did research on restorative herbs and minerals, as well as selling those products to local residents (Giovannini and Mancini 1987). At almost the same time, 1220, the first educational institution devoted exclusively to the training of physicians opened in Montpellier, France: the Univeratas Medicorum. The school continues in operation today (Régnier 2020).

Over the centuries, the field of pharmaceutics continued to grow and develop in essentially the same way as did other professions. For example, in 1617, King James I of England created the Society of Apothecaries. Over time, the society grew in power until, by 1815, it had become responsible for the control of all forms of medical practice in Great Britain (Copeman 1967). The pharmaceutical profession followed a similar line of development in the United States. The first institution for training pharmacists was founded in 1821, the Philadelphia College of Apothecaries. The school was formed largely because of growing concerns about the lack of training and generally poor practice of pharmaceutics in the United States. The college became part of the University of Pennsylvania, which granted the first master of pharmacy degrees in 1821, even though none of the recipients had actually studied at Penn

("Announcement of the Founding of the Philadelphia College of Pharmacy" 2008).

As in Great Britain, and throughout history, many individuals involved in the pharmaceutical industry were concerned about its reputation because of unethical practices by some practitioners. In response to that concern, representatives from a group of local and regional pharmaceutical groups met in Pennsylvania to form the American Pharmaceutical Association, which continues to exist today as the American Pharmacists Association.

Narcotics

One recurring problem throughout the history of medicine centers on one specific group of compounds: narcotics. As noted previously, the traditional meaning for the term *narcotics* is any compound that affects a person's mood or behavior, often when it is used for nonmedical purposes. Today, most authorities restrict the use of the term to an even more specific group of compounds: the opioids. An opioid is a derivative or semi-synthetic product of naturally occurring opium. The most common opioids in use today are codeine, fentanyl, heroin, hydrocodone, morphine. oxycodone, and tramadol.

Probably the earliest date for which narcotics are known might be about 5000 BCE. One study has reported on seeds of the ephedra plant that even today is used for its psychoactive effects. The problem with such data is that natural products will have degraded so badly over that period of time that one cannot be sure that the ancient plant is the same as the modern plant and if the compound was used for medical purposes, recreational purposes, or both. Most commonly, the earliest date for the use of narcotics is about 3400 BCE. Records from that period of time in Sumeria refer to a plant known as *hul gil*, or "joy plant." That nomenclature suggests (but does not prove) that the plant, a form of the opium poppy, was used for recreational purposes (Krikorian 1975).

Over time, knowledge, cultivation, and use of opium was handed down from the Mesopotamians to the Phoenicians, Minoans, and Egyptians. Our first certain knowledge of its cultivation dates to about 1300 BCE, when the poppy plant was cultivated in the area around Thebes, capital of Egypt at the time. Often cited as perhaps the most striking surviving evidence of the place of opium in Middle Eastern civilizations is the so-called poppy goddess from the island of Crete, also in about 1300 BCE. This terra cotta figure of a women includes a crown of flower buds that are almost certainly capsules of the poppy plant. Many authorities have argued that the figure confirms the use of opium in meditative or other mind-altering experiences in early Minoan civilization (Bowen 2013).

Throughout the pre-Christian era in the Middle East, Asia, Europe, and other regions, opium was an important part of the healer's collection of tools in dealing with disease and injury. The most important of these applications made use of the compound's soporific (sleep inducing) and analgesic (pain reducing) properties. For example, the great Greek physician Hippocrates recommended the use of poppy derivatives for a wide variety of disorders but generally dismissed the usefulness of its psychoactive or other nonphysical uses (Kritikos and Papadaki 1967).

In some ways, the most dramatic element in the history of opium use began in the early sixteenth century, when Portuguese merchants trading along the coasts of India learned about opium and developed the practice of smoking the drug for its narcotic effects. These travelers soon exported the practice to China, where the drug had long been held in disrepute, and to England, where its medical value was well known. The effort to force Chinese officials to accept the importation of opium to their country by British ships eventually led to a series of conflicts known as the Opium Wars. The two wars, one from 1839 to 1842, and the other, from 1856 to 1860, led to the defeat of the Chinese military and the nation's acceptance of shipments of opium to its shores (Hanes and Sanello 2002).

Meanwhile, physicians, pharmacists, early chemists, and other researchers were beginning to learn more scientific and technical information about opium. Among the first of these breakthroughs was the invention in 1527 of an elixir known as *laudanum*. An *elixir* is a liquid solution in which a medicine is made more palatable by the addition of a substance or substances with a pleasant flavor. When the solvent used is an alcohol, the mixture is known as a *tincture*. The product was invented by Swiss physician Theophrastus von Hohenheim (generally known as Paracelsus). Given the secrecy of such work at the time, we do not know the precise composition of Paracelsus's laudanum, although it is thought to have consisted of opium, alcohol, gold leaf, pearls, and other substances (Sigerist 1941).

For over a century, Paracelsus's laudanum was an essential part of the materia medica used by most physicians in the Western world. Then, in 1680, English apothecary Thomas Sydenham devised a new and better recipe for laudanum. Sydenham's laudanum consisted of 1 gram of opium dissolved in 100 milliliters of alcohol. The preparation was made more palatable with the addition of species such as cinnamon, clover, and saffron. Sydenham's enthusiasm for the product is reflected in what is perhaps his most famous quote on the topic: "Of all the remedies it has pleased almighty God to give man to relieve his suffering," he once wrote, "none is so universal and so efficacious as opium" (Inglis 2019, 124–133).

During the nineteenth century, laudanum became particularly popular among some of the best-known writers and artists of the age. Some used it primarily or at least originally for the treatment of pain or some other condition. But in many cases, an individual used the drug solely for recreational purposes, often claiming that its effect transported a person above and beyond the clutter of everyday life. Among the Victorian personages who used, became addicted to, or even died from the use of laudanum were Elizabeth Barrett Browning, Lord Byron, Wilkie Collins, Samuel Taylor Coleridge, Charles Dickens, Sir

Arthur Conan Doyle, George Eliot, Elizabeth Gaskell, John Keats, Edgar Allan Poe, Gabriel Dante Rossetti, and his wife Elizabeth Siddal (who died from an opium overdose), Percy Bysshe Shelley, and Bram Stoker (Diniejko 2002, Milligan 2003).

Laudanum was also "the drug of choice" among many ordinary individuals. It was, first of all, easy to obtain. All one had to do was to walk into the nearest pharmacy to purchase a bottle, usually at a very modest price. No prescription or formal monitoring of any kind was necessary. The drug was especially popular among young mothers, as a way of quieting crying babies. Since the tincture also provided users with a buzz, it also became popular among workers or the unemployed whose life had been made especially difficult by the advent of the Industrial Revolution. For these reasons, laudanum is often called "the aspirin of the nineteenth century" (Diniejko 2002).

In the United States, laudanum was also readily available, often a component of the so-called patent medicines that were so widely popular in the nineteenth century. Patent medicines are medicines made under a patent that can be sold "over the counter" without prescription (Brecher and the Editors of Consumers Reports 1972, O'Neill 2012). Laudanum has now been banned in most countries, although it is still available by prescription in the United States, where it is a Schedule II drug.

Opiates

The next great step forward in the study of opium came in 1803, when German chemist Friedrich Wilhelm Adam Sertürner discovered morphine. At the time, the field of chemistry was in its earliest stages of discovery, and the chemical nature of natural products was a virtually unknown topic. It never occurred to most chemists of the time that plants and animals might have chemical compositions as do minerals and other nonliving materials. So Sertürner's discovery marked an important step forward not only for the study of opium but also for the field of chemistry in general. Morphine is now considered to be the first *opiate* drug discovered after opium itself. An opiate drug is a naturally occurring drug obtained from the poppy plant *Papaver somniferum*. Opiates are now considered to be a sub-category of *opioids*, compounds that have psychoactive effects like those of the opiates but not obtained from *P. somniferum* and with different chemical structures.

Sertürner made his discovery by carrying out some of the simplest possible chemical reactions one can imagine. He dissolved some opium powder in hot water and then added ammonia to the mixture. He found that a white precipitate (solid) settled out of the solution, a new compound to which he gave the name *morphine*. He chose that name when he found that ingestion of the compound caused an animal to become sleepy: Morpheus was recognized by the ancient Greeks as the god of sleep.

Sertürner's earliest research on morphine was troubling, to say the least. He tested the compound on a mouse, three dogs, three young boys, and himself. The mouse and dogs died, and the four humans all became gravely ill. When Sertürner wrote a scholarly paper describing his work, he emphasized these dangerous effects in the paper's title: *Ueber eins der Fürchterlichsten Gifte der Pflanzenwelt* ("About One of the Most Terrible Poisons of the Plant World"). (Sertürner's original paper is available, in German, at Sertürner 1817.)

In spite of the negative effects Sertürner observed for his new discovery, he decided to form a firm to market the drug to the general public. That enterprise was not successful, however, for two reasons. One was the complexity of the procedure for making the compound, and the other was the lack of an efficient way to introduce morphine into the human body. The first of these problems was solved in 1831, when Scottish chemist William Gregory discovered a more efficient way to produce the drug. The second problem disappeared with the invention of the hypodermic needle by Scottish physicist Alexander Wood in 1853. These developments made it possible to begin manufacturing and selling morphine to the general

Table 1.4 Naturally Occurring Opioids

Opiate	Year	Discoverer	Reference
Noscapine (also narcotine and other synonyms)	803	Jean-François Derosne	Padmashree, et al. 2015
Codeine	832	Pierre-Jean Robiquet	Wisniak 2013
Narceine	832	Pierre-Joseph Pelletier	Pelletier 2020
Thebaine	835	Pierre-Joseph Pelletier and Thibouméry	Small 1932
Papaverine	848	Georg Merck	Harrison 2013

public, a step first taken by the young Merck pharmaceutical company in Germany in 1827 ("Pharmaceutical Research by a Commercial House" 1906). Five years later in the United States, a relatively young new pharmaceutical firm, Zeitler and Rosengarten, began manufacturing opium products also, shortly becoming the world's largest producer of morphine (The Powers-Weightman-Rosengarten Company 1925).

The 1830s and 1840s were a very rich period for opium chemistry. Several research groups carried out variations of Sertürner's experiments on opium, discovering a half dozen new compounds present in the opium plant in small quantities. Table 1.4 summarizes these naturally occurring opiates, with information about their discovery.

Semi-Synthetic Opioids

From their earliest discoveries, the opiates presented medical workers and researchers with contrasting issues. On the one hand, these compounds obviously had the potential to be powerful elements in the medical arsenal against disease and injury. They were much stronger painkillers than any existing compounds available for that purpose. On the other hand, opiates also had serious drawbacks. In addition to the adverse reactions observed by Sertürner, it soon became obvious that they readily led to dependence and addiction. As is the case throughout the history of medicine, researchers' response to this conundrum was to begin looking for new compounds, from either natural sources or the results of laboratory research, that were at least as powerful as opiates and much safer to use. The obvious approach for much of this research was to find ways of manipulating the opium molecule so as to change its chemical structure and, thereby, its psychoactive effects. Such compounds became known as *semi-synthetic opioids*, "semi-synthetic" because they were actually made in a chemical laboratory and "opioids" because they sometimes had structures similar to the structure of opium but always had similar psychoactive effects.

The first breakthrough in the search for semi-synthetic forms of the opiates occurred at St. Mary's Hospital in London in 1874. C. R. Alder Wright, a chemist working at the hospital, was trying a variety of modifications of the morphine molecule to see if he could solve at least one of the two problems described previously. In one of these attempts, he added two acetyl groups to the morphine molecule, producing a new substance called *diacetylmorphine* or *morphine diacetate*. A comparison of the molecular structure of morphine and heroin is available at "Opium, Morphine, and Heroin" (2015).

Wright sent a sample of his product to a colleague, F. M. Pierce, for testing on animals. Pierce described the effect of the substance on young dogs and rabbits that were injected with it. The most noticeable effects, Pierce said, were

> great prostration, fear, and sleepiness speedily following the administration, the eyes being sensitive, and pupils dilated, considerable salivation being produced in dogs, and slight tendency to vomiting in some cases, but no actual emesis. Respiration was [at] first quickened, but subsequently reduced, and the heart's action was diminished, and rendered irregular. Marked want of co-ordinating power over the muscular movements, and loss of power in the pelvis and hind limbs, together with a diminution of temperature in the rectum of about 4°. (Wright 1874, 1043)

These results may at least partly account for the fact that Wright went no further with his research on diacetylmorphine, a substance that attracted no attention for more than twenty years. Then, in 1897, a researcher at the Aktiengesellschaft Farbenfabriken pharmaceutical company (later to become the giant pharmaceutical manufacturer Bayer), Felix Hoffmann, turned his attention to the same line of research as that pursued by Wright. He rediscovered essentially the same chemical and pharmacological properties as those observed by Wright and Pierce but also saw the marketing potential for the new drug. Heroin was about twice as efficacious as morphine, and it appeared at first to have none of the addictive properties of the natural opiate. Aktiengesellschaft Farbenfabriken began an aggressive advertising campaign for their new product (named *heroin*, after the German word *heroisch*, for "heroic") based on its efficacy and safety. It was recommended as a substitute for morphine and used as a constituent in cough syrups. In perhaps its most optimistic recommendation, the company even suggested that heroin could be used to wean morphine addicts off the natural opiate, a claim that very quickly turned out to be not true (Durlacher 2000).

Over the next half century, researchers discovered about a half dozen semi-synthetic opioids with therapeutic value (and, often, harmful side effects). The first of these drugs, oxymorphone, was discovered in Germany in about 1914 but not made available in the United States until 1959. It is made from the opium constituent thebaine. A second semi-synthetic opioid, oxycodone, was also produced in Germany two years later by chemists Martin Freund and Edmund Speyer. Oxycodone was also first made from thebaine and became available in the United States in 1939. Hydrocodone was first prepared in 1920 by German chemists Carl Mannich and Helene Löwenheim. The drug was marketed by the pharmaceutical firm Knoll four years later under the name Dicodid. It was approved for sale in the United States in 1943. Both hydrocodone and oxycodone are derivatives of codeine.

Hydromorphone was first synthesized in 1924, also by researchers at Knoll, which marketed the drug under the name Dilaudid two years later. Hydromorphone is a derivative of morphine, synthesized by adding hydrogen to one of the ketone groups in morphine. Etorphine was first produced in 1960. Its synthesis is somewhat unusual in that it is made from oripavine, a constituent of opium poppy straw, rather than from the poppy seed itself. Etorphine is up to 3,000 times as strong as morphine and is currently legal in the United States only for veterinary uses. The discovery of buprenorphine was announced in 1972 as the result of a targeted research program at the Reckitt & Coleman pharmaceutical company (now Reckitt Benckiser) to find a safer version of heroin. The most important use of buprenorphine today is for the treatment of addiction to other opioids. For a good general introduction to semi-synthetic opioids, see "Semi-Synthetic Opioids" (n.d.).

Synthetic Opioids

The search for safe and efficacious opioids in the mid-twentieth century also focused on completely synthetic compounds, that is, compounds created from non-opium materials such as coal tar and other petroleum products. The first such compound discovered was pethidine, developed by German chemist Otto Eisleb (also given as Eislib) in 1932. Eislib was originally looking for an anticholinergic medication (one that treats disorders of the gastrointestinal system) and was not aware of its analgesic effects. Those effects were later discovered by another German chemist, Otto Schaumann, in 1939. The drug was later given the generic name meperdine and sold under the trade name Dolantin. It is now known as Demerol and listed as a Schedule II drug by the DEA (Hori and Gold 1944).

Another synthetic opioid of some significance developed in the late 1930s was methadone. The drug was developed by German researchers at the pharmaceutical laboratories of the

I. G. Farbenkonzern company. It was one of many drugs that were being tested as analgesics in preparation for the demands of World War II injuries. Originally called Compound Va10820, the drug was officially named methadone in 1947 by the Council on Pharmacy and Chemistry of the American Medical Association. Methadone has been used both for its analgesic properties and as an effective therapy for withdrawal from addiction to more dangerous opiates and opioids (Gerlach 2004).

Research on synthetic opioids has been one of the most consequential topics in the field of pharmaceutical drugs in at least the past two decades. On the one hand, legitimate researchers continue the ages-old search for drugs with improved therapeutic properties to be used in all fields of medicine. On the other hand, unlawful researchers are constantly trying to develop opioid drugs that can be used for illegal, recreational purposes. The battle has been, then, between governmental agencies attempting to monitor and control the development and distribution of dangerous opioid products and illicit manufacturers constantly trying to bring new and non-Scheduled drugs to the market for addicts and other abusers of drugs. Almost as soon as a new synthetic opioid is discovered, it is studied and listed on the DEA Schedule. For example, as soon as the dangers of the synthetic drug fentanyl were discovered and it was listed as a Schedule II drug, analogs ("substantially similar") were developed and also scheduled by the DEA. Some fentanyl analogs currently listed by the DEA are 3-methylfentayl, 3-methylthiofentanyl, despropionylfentanyl, 4-fluoroisobutyrylfentanyl, acetylfentanyl, acetyl-alpha-methylfentanyl, acrylfentanyl, alpha-methylthiofentanyl, beta-hydroxy-3-methylfentanyl, and on and on ("Controlled Substances" 2020); for more details on the current status of semi-synthetic and synthetic drugs in the United States, see "2019 National Drug Threat Assessment" (2019) and "Synthetic Opioids: The Ugly and Deadly Truth" (2020).

Monitoring of Drug Use

The second half of the nineteenth century was a time of considerable turmoil for the medical profession in the United States and elsewhere in the world. Several new drugs had been invented or discovered to treat medical conditions, especially pain, more effectively than anything previously available. People suffering from cancer, for example, had for the first time ever drugs stronger than aspirin to treat their recurring pain and discomfort. Even the everyday housewife with six children was able to achieve a modicum of relief with a drop of opium on the crying baby's tongue.

But these new "wonder drugs," such as laudanum and morphine, were certainly not unalloyed blessings. They brought with them new challenges both for the medical profession itself and for the general populace. Most disturbing, perhaps, was the fact that *anyone* could call herself or himself a "healer" and set up a "medical practice" for treating a host of medical conditions. No license was need, nor were there any kinds of standards to which the purveyor of a "medicine" had to attend. As a result, untold numbers of "healers" set up business in a downtown shop, on a dusty rural trail, or in any other imaginable setting. There they could make available to largely uneducated crowds medications such as laudanum and morphine for the cure not only of pain but of a seemingly endless list of medical conditions. One product, for example, Hostetter's Celebrated Stomach Bitters, claimed a range of benefits, including "dyspepsia, liver complaint, costiveness and indigestion, intermittent fever, fever and ague, a good anti-bilious, powerful recuperant, appetizer, strengthener of digestive forces, corrective and mild cathartic" ("Balm of America: Patent Medicine Collection" n.d., which lists a good selection of patent medicines). The popularity of these medications depended partly on the fact that they sometimes did help a person's suffering, but it was not harmed by the fact that such "patent medicines" often contained significant concentrations of alcohol (Young 1961/2015).

By the last quarter of the nineteenth century, legislators were beginning to appreciate the scope of the patent medicine problem. That problem was closely related to another important issue: the adulteration of food. Many food purveyors routinely added foreign substances to foods to increase their profit in the sale of such materials. For example, chalk was often added to milk to reduce the amount of product (milk) for some given price (Hart 1952). The earliest effort by Congress to deal with this problem came in 1879, when Representative Hendrick Bradley Wright introduced a bill to prevent the adulteration of food. The bill was never reported out of committee. A year later, however, additional bills were introduced, four of which related to the adulteration of drugs. None of those bills advanced beyond committee either (Wilson 1942). Bills dealing with the regulation of foods and drugs were routinely introduced in each session of Congress over the next twenty-seven years. Finally, in 1906, Congress passed the Pure Food and Drugs Act, the law that still forms the basis for the regulation of foods and drugs in the United States (Barkan 1985).

The Pure Food and Drugs Act did not, by any stretch of imagination, resolve issues surrounding the use of narcotic drugs in the United States and some other countries. Of particular concern was the diversion of opium, laudanum, and morphine to nonmedical uses, such as recreational smoking. That concern blossomed in 1898 with the annexation of the Philippine Islands by the United States. Of special concern to religious leaders at the time was the opium industry operated by the Philippine government itself. Charles Henry Brent, Episcopalian bishop of the Islands at the time, prevailed upon a group of friends with similar concerns to petition President Theodore Roosevelt to call for an international conference to design a system for monitoring the illegal use of opiates. (The conference later added another narcotic drug, cocaine, to this agenda.) This international conference, thus, was originally driven by and strongly influenced by religious leaders with concerns about illegal drug use, with relatively minor contributions from scientific experts in the field.

The Shanghai Conference became only the first of a series of international meetings on the control of opiates, cocaine, marijuana (added at the last moment of the Shanghai meeting), and other narcotics. Today, three of those meetings in particular form the basis for an international system of monitoring and control of narcotic drugs: the Single Convention on Narcotic Drugs (1961), the Convention on Psychotropic Substances (1971), and the Convention against Illicit Traffic in Narcotic Drugs and Psychotropic Substances (1988) (Sinha 2001).

Somewhat remarkably, almost no specific legislation dealing with the prescribing of drugs was adopted in the United States prior to 1951. One interesting exception to that statement occurred during the period of Prohibition in the United States, between 1920 and 1933. During that period, the purchase of alcoholic beverages was prohibited in the country. But a special provision of Prohibition's enabling legislation, the Volstead Act, allowed physicians to write prescriptions for "medicinal alcohol," alcohol used to treat medical conditions. Some doctors took that exception quite generously, writing prescriptions for conditions ranging from old age, diabetes, asthma, cancer, and anemia to rheumatism, snake bite, problems of pregnancy, and insomnia (Jones 1963, Mejia 2017).

A key development in federal regulations about prescription drugs came with the adoption of the Federal Food, Drug, and Cosmetic Act of 1938 (FD&C). There had been considerable debate over the safety of drugs for consumer use throughout the first third of the twentieth century. But legislative bodies tended to take little action for dealing with that issue. That situation changed in 1937, when more than one hundred patients in the United States died from ingestion of the drug elixir sulfanilamide. The drug had previously been used for the treatment of streptococcal and similar infections with apparently satisfactory success. As it developed, the drug also had serious side effects that had resulted in the wave of deaths reported in fifteen states in 1937. That event was largely responsible for the passage of the FD&C a year later. That law, for the first time in U.S. history, established procedures to ensure that any drug offered for human use in the country would first have to be proved safe for that purpose. No regulation was provided, however, for ensuring the efficacy of a drug (Ballentine 1981).

The issue of drug efficacy remained in limbo for more than a decade after adoption of the FD&C. Then, in 1951, Congress adopted the Durham-Humphrey Amendment to the FD&C, a piece of legislation that has become the defining document for prescription drugs in the United States. One provision of the Act provided, for the first time, a clear distinction between prescription and over-the-counter drugs. The former were defined as drugs that might tend to addiction and/or be harmful to human health. The application of the distinction between the two categories for any particular product was left up to drug manufacturers, although the FDA could deny a license to any drug that met the conditions noted here. The Act also required the use of a "label" for any prescription drug that included information such as name and address of the pharmacy supplying the product, serial number of the prescription, date of its filling, name of the prescriber, name of the patient, the directions for use, and any applicable warning labels. Arguably, the most important single feature of the law was the requirement that the following statement be included on every prescription drug label: "Caution: Federal law prohibits dispensing without a prescription" ("Public Law 215. Chapter 578" 1951); for a full discussion of the Durham-Humphrey Amendment, see Reilly (2006).

More recent prescription drug legislation has developed largely in response to specific issues that developed within the field. For example, by the mid-1980s, it had become apparent that avenues had developed through which untested and/or unapproved drugs could be provided for sale to the U.S. public. For example, an offshore company might purchase drugs from a U.S. manufacturer and then repackage them and sell them to U.S. consumers. Provisions in place for ensuring the safety of drugs would thus be defeated by this process. To deal with problems of this kind, Congress passed the Prescription Drug Marketing Act of 1988 (Sasich 2000).

Another piece of federal legislation, the Medicare Prescription Drug Improvement and Modernization Act (also known as the Medicare Modernization Act or, simply, MMA), was adopted in 2003. That law was driven by the fact that relatively few changes had been made to the original Medicare Act of 1965 that provided essential health care for most Americans. In the decades following its adoption, the cost of prescription drugs had increased substantially, so that many individuals, especially senior citizens, were unable to afford even the most basic drugs needed to maintain their health.

Perhaps the most important provision of that long and complex Act was the creation of a new category of Medicare coverage, originally called Part D (as an addition to existing Parts A, B, and C of the program). This section provided systems by which senior citizens could obtain prescription drugs at discounts of at least 10 percent over normal prices. One element of that system was a drug discount card available to all seniors and certain other individuals with disabilities. Presentation of that card at a pharmacy resulted in a discount on the cost of drugs purchased at that pharmacy. According to one estimate, the average senior could save as much as $300 on an annual cost of $1,285 for prescription drugs ("Fact Sheet: Medicare Prescription Drug, Improvement, and Modernization Act of 2003" 2003); a much more detailed summary of this complex law may be found at "H.R.1—Medicare Prescription Drug, Improvement, and Modernization Act of 2003" (2003).

Another issue of growing concern in the field of prescription drugs has been the sale of such products online. Today, it is often possible to find websites from which an individual can purchase drugs that are normally prescription products. Among the most popular of these products are narcotics that can be used for recreational as well as medicinal purposes. Several websites on the so-called dark web advertise such products, which can be purchased either without a prescription or with a prescription provided by an illegal health provider (Hill 2019). In an effort to deal with this problem, the U.S. Congress in 2008 adopted the Ryan Haight Online Pharmacy Consumer Protection Act. The most important provision of that Act is the requirement that controlled substances cannot be delivered, distributed, or dispensed without a valid prescription. In addition, such a prescription cannot be written without there having first been a face-to-face meeting between the patient and a qualified medical provider ("Telemedicine Prescribing of Controlled Substances: What Is the Ryan Haight Act?" 2017). A good overall review of the history of federal prescription drug legislation is available at "Milestones in U.S. Food and Drug Law History" (2018).

In addition to federal legislation dealing with prescription drugs, almost all states have adopted a variety of laws to deal with some specific aspects of the field. Among the most common of those state laws are those dealing with prescription drug monitoring programs (PDMPs) and doctor shopping laws. Both types of law are intended to reduce the problem of prescription drug abuse, that is, the use of such drugs for recreational purposes for individuals for whom they are normally not prescribed. (This topic is discussed further in Chapter 2.) A PDMP is an electronic database that has records of prescriptions written for controlled substances, such as opioids, along with the names of prescribers and individuals for whom a prescription has been written. When a health care worker decides to write a prescription for a person, the worker can check the database for that individual's prescription history, reducing the risk of having that individual overprescribed. When a prescription is filled, a pharmacist enters relevant information about the transaction in the database, providing the basic information needed by the caregiver ("Prescription Drug Monitoring Programs [PDMPs]" 2020); a sample PDMP law is given in Chapter 5. As of late 2020, forty-nine states, the District of Columbia, and Guam had PDMP laws. Only Missouri had not yet adopted such a law, although lobbying for such a law has been going on for many years (Jason 2020).

The term *doctor shopping* refers to a practice common among prescription drug abusers. It involves an individual's visiting several health care professionals in order to obtain the prescription drugs the individual needs to maintain a drug abuse habit. Such a practice has been illegal according to federal laws since the adoption of the Uniform Narcotic Drug Act of 1932. The Act specifies that "no person shall obtain or attempt to obtain a narcotic drug, or procure or attempt to procure the administration of a narcotic drug . . . by fraud, deceit, misrepresentation, or subterfuge or . . . by the concealment of a material fact" ("Doctor Shopping Laws" 2012). As of 2020, all fifty states have doctor shopping laws that include exactly or almost precisely this wording. In addition to these federal regulations, many states have adopted discreet, standalone laws prohibiting doctor shopping and providing specific penalties for such activities. As of late 2020, twenty-three states had some form of this additional regulation (Nenn 2019); a sample doctor shopping law is reproduced in Chapter 5.

Conclusion

The history of prescription drug development over the ages provides, on the one hand, an encouraging story about the constant search for and discovery of new products that can be used to treat disease and injuries in humans and animals. In that sense, the story of prescription drugs is one of constant progress and improvement. On the other hand, almost every step in the timeline of prescription drug development has been accompanied by the appearance of some type of technical, social, political, economic, or health problem. That has been the case since the earliest known appearance of mind-altering drugs such as opium to the most recent challenge of finding ways to make prescription drugs available to those who need them at some level of reasonable cost. A more detailed study of some of these problems and possible solutions is the subject of Chapter 2.

References

Ajami, Alfred, and Andrii Buvailo. 2017. "36 Web Resources for Target Hunting in Drug Discovery." https://www .biopharmatrend.com/post/45-27-web-resources-for-target-hunting-in-drug-discovery/.

"Announcement of the Founding of the Philadelphia College of Pharmacy." 2008. *Pharmacy in History*. 50(1): 27–29.

Ballentine, Carol. 1981. "Sulfanilamide Disaster." *FDA Consumer*. https://www.fda.gov/files/about%20fda/ published/The-Sulfanilamide-Disaster.pdf.

"Balm of America: Patent Medicine Collection." n.d. National Museum of American History. https:// americanhistory.si.edu/collections/object-groups/ balm-of-america-patent-medicine-collection.

Barkan, Ilyse D. 1985. "Industry Invites Regulation: The Passage of the Pure Food and Drug Act of 1906." *American Journal of Public Health*. 75(1): 18–26. https://ajph .aphapublications.org/doi/pdf/10.2105/AJPH.75.1.18.

"Biopharmaceutical Research & Development: The Process Behind New Medicines." 2015. PHRMA. http:// phrma-docs.phrma.org/sites/default/files/pdf/rd_ brochure_022307.pdf.

Bowen, Monica. 2013. "Minoans, the 'Poppy Goddess' and Opium." Alberti's Window. http://albertis-window .com/2013/10/minoans-the-poppy-goddess-and-opium/.

Brecher, Edward M., and the Editors of Consumer Reports. 1972. *Licit and Illicit Drugs*. Boston, Toronto: Little, Brown. http://www.druglibrary.org/schaffer/library/studies/ cu/cumenu.htm.

Carroll, John. 2017. "The List of the Top 10 Most Expensive Drugs on the Planet Will Soon Have a New Opening." Endpoint News. https://endpts.com/the-list-of-the-top-10-most-expensive-drugs-on-the-planet-will-soon-have-a-new-opening/.

"Category Names, Results, and Descriptions." 2020. Drug Information Portal. U.S. National Library of Medicine. https://druginfo.nlm.nih.gov/drugportal/drug/categories.

"Chapter XIII—Requirements for Informed Consent." n.d. Genetic Alliance. http://geneticalliance.org/chapter-xiii-requirements-informed-consent.

"ClinCalc DrugStats Database." 2021. https://clincalc.com/DrugStats/.

"Controlled Substances." 2020. [Drug Enforcement Agency]. https://www.deadiversion.usdoj.gov/schedules/orangebook/c_cs_alpha.pdf.

"The Controlled Substances Act." n.d. U.S. Drug Enforcement Administration. https://www.dea.gov/controlled-substances-act.

Copeman, W. S. C. 1967. *The Worshipful Society of Apothecaries of London: A History, 1617–1967*. Oxford: Pergamon Press.

Davidson, Tish. 2019. *The Vaccine Debate*. Santa Barbara, CA: Greenwood.

Desborough, Michael J. R., and David M. Keeling. 2017. "The Aspirin Story—From Willow to Wonder Drug." *British Journal of Haematology*. 177(5): 674–683. https://onlinelibrary.wiley.com/doi/pdf/10.1111/bjh.14520.

"Developing Products for Rare Diseases & Conditions." 2018. U.S. Food and Drug Administration. https://www.fda.gov/industry/developing-products-rare-diseases-conditions.

Diniejko, Andrzej. 2002. "Victorian Drug Use." The Victorian Web. http://www.victorianweb.org/victorian/science/addiction/addiction2.html.

"Doctor Shopping Laws." 2012. Centers for Disease Control and Prevention. http://www.cdc.gov/phlp/docs/menu-shoppinglaws.pdf.

"Drugs@FDA Glossary of Terms." 2017. U.S. Food and Drug Administration. https://www.fda.gov/drugs/drug-approvals-and-databases/drugsfda-glossary-terms

Durlacher, Julian. 2000. *Heroin: Its History and Lore*. London: Carlton Books.

"Fact Sheet: Medicare Prescription Drug, Improvement, and Modernization Act of 2003." 2003. The White House. https://georgewbush-whitehouse.archives.gov/news/releases/2003/12/20031208-3.html.

Fisher, Jill A., and Corey A. Kalbaugh. 2011. "Challenging Assumptions about Minority Participation in US Clinical Research." *American Journal of Public Health*. 101(12): 2217–2222. doi: 10.2105/AJPH.2011.300279.

Gerlach, Ralf. 2004. "The History of Methadone." Indo e.V. https://indro-online.de/en/the-history-of-methadone/.

Giovannini, Sandra, and Gabriella Mancini. 1987. *The Pharmacy of Santa Maria Novella*. Florence: Becocci.

"Guidance for FDA Staff and Industry." 2011. Center for Drug Evaluation and Research, U.S. Food and Drug Administration. https://www.fda.gov/media/71004/download.

Hanes, William Travis, and Frank Sanello. 2002. *The Opium Wars: The Addiction of One Empire and the Corruption of Another*. London: Robson.

Hanneman, Joe. 2014. "The History of Pharmacy by Artist Robert Thom." Hanneman Archive. https://hannemanarchive.com/2014/12/12/history-of-pharmacy/.

Harrison, Karl. 2013. "Papaverine (Molecule of the Month for February 2013)." 3DChem.com. http://www.3dchem.com/Papaverine.asp.

Hart, F. Leslie. 1952. "A History of the Adulteration of Food Before 1906." *Food, Drug, Cosmetic Law Journal.* 7(1): 5–22. https://www.jstor.org/stable/26654178.

Hefti, Franz F. 2008. "Requirements for a Lead Compound to Become a Clinical Candidate." *BMC Neuroscience.* 9(Suppl 3): S7. doi: 10.1186/1471-2202-9-S3-S7.

Hill, Stef. 2019. "Doctor Google and the Dark Web Pharmacist." Medium. https://medium.com/@Stefanina Hill/doctor-google-and-the-dark-web-pharmacist-1acd657ffe2f.

Hori, C. George, and Simon Gold. 1944. "Demerol in Surgery and Obstetrics." *Canadian Medical Association Journal.* 51(6): 509–517. https://www.ncbi.nlm.nih.gov/pmc/articles/PMC1582053/.

"H.R.1—Medicare Prescription Drug, Improvement, and Modernization Act of 2003." 2003. Congress.gov. https://www.congress.gov/bill/108th-congress/house-bill/1.

Hughes, J. P., et al. 2011. "Principles of Early Drug Discovery." *British Journal of Pharmacology.* 162(6): 1239–1249. doi: 10.1111/j.1476-5381.2010.01127.x.

Inglis, Lucy. 2019. *Milk of Paradise.* New York: Pegasus Books.

"Investigational New Drug Application." 2020. U.S. Food and Drug Administration. https://www.fda.gov/drugs/types-applications/investigational-new-drug-ind-application.

Jason, Christopher. 2020. "MO May Be Final State to Tap Prescription Drug Monitoring Program." EHR Intelligence. https://ehrintelligence.com/news/mo-may-be-final-state-to-tap-prescription-drug-monitoring-program.

Jones, Bartlett C. 1963. "A Prohibition Problem: Liquor as Medicine, 1920–1933." *Journal of the History of Medicine and Allied Sciences.* 18(4): 353–369.

Khan, Ikhlas A., and Ehab A. Abourashed. 2013. *Leung's Encyclopedia of Common Natural Ingredients Used in Food, Drugs and Cosmetics*, 3rd ed. Hoboken, NJ: Wiley.

Kremers, Edward, George Urdang, and Glenn Sonnedecker. 1976/1986. *Kremers and Urdang's History of Pharmacy.* Madison, WI: American Institute of the History of Pharmacy.

Krikorian, Abraham D. 1975. "Were the Opium Poppy and Opium Known in the Ancient near East?" *Journal of the History of Biology.* 8(1): 95–114.

Kritikos, P. G., and S. P. Papadaki. 1967. "The History of the Poppy and of Opium and Their Expansion in Antiquity in the Eastern Mediterranean Area." United Nations Office on Drugs and Crime. https://www.unodc.org/unodc/en/data-and-analysis/bulletin/bulletin_1967-01-01_3_page004.html.

Kummar, Shivaani, et al. 2008. "Phase 0 Clinical Trials: Conceptions and Misconceptions." *Cancer Journal.* 14(3): 133–137. doi: 10.1097/PPO.0b013e318172d6f3.

Lal, Renu, and Mary Kremzner. 2017. "Introduction to the New Prescription Drug Labeling by the Food and Drug Administration." *American Journal of Health–System Pharmacy.* 64(23): 2488–2494. doi.org/10.2146/ajhp070130.

"List of Vaccines Used in the United States." 2018. Centers for Disease Control and Prevention. https://www.cdc.gov/vaccines/vpd/vaccines-list.html.

Mejia, Paula. 2017. "The Lucrative Business of Prescribing Booze During Prohibition." Atlas Obscura. https://www.atlasobscura.com/articles/doctors-booze-notes-prohibition.

"Milestones in U.S. Food and Drug Law History." 2018. U.S. Food and Drug Administration. https://www.fda.gov/about-fda/fdas-evolving-regulatory-powers/milestones-us-food-and-drug-law-history.

Milligan, Barry. 2003. *Confessions of an Opium Eater. Thomas De Quincey*. London: Penguin Books.

"Narcotics (Opioids)." n.d. U.S. Drug Enforcement Administration. https://www.dea.gov/taxonomy/term/331.

Nenn, Kerry. 2019. "Here's What You Need to Know about Doctor Shopping." National Rehabs Directory. https://www.rehabs.com/blog/heres-what-you-need-to-know-about-doctor-shopping/.

"New Drug Application (NDA)." 2019. U.S. Food and Drug Administration. https://www.fda.gov/drugs/types-applications/new-drug-application-nda.

"Off-Label Drug Prescribing: What Does It Mean for You?" 2015. Consumer Reports. https://www.consumerreports.org/cro/2012/05/off-label-drug-prescribing-what-does-it-mean-for-you/index.htm.

O'Neill, Tony. 2012. "10 Old-Timey Medicines That Got People High." Alternet. https://www.alternet.org/drugs/10-old-timey-medicines-got-people-high.

"Opium, Morphine, and Heroin." 2015. http://www.ch.ic.ac.uk/rzepa/mim/drugs/html/morphine_text.htm.

Osborn, David K. 2018. "Dioscorides." Greek Medicine. http://www.greekmedicine.net/whos_who/Dioscorides.html.

"OTC Drug Facts Label." 2015. U.S. Food and Drug Administration. https://www.fda.gov/drugs/drug-information-consumers/otc-drug-facts-label.

Padmashree, C. G. Rida, et al. 2015. "The Noscapine Chronicle: A Pharmaco-Historic Biography of the Opiate Alkaloid Family and Its Clinical Applications." *Medicinal Research Reviews*. 35(5): 1072–1096. doi: 10.1002/med.21357.

Peckham, Alyssa M., et al. 2018. "Gabapentin for Off-Label Use: Evidence-Based or Cause for Concern?"

Substance Abuse: Research and Treatment. doi: 10.1177/1178221818801311.

Pelletier, Pierre-Joseph. 2020. "Encyclopedia Britannica." https://www.britannica.com/biography/Pierre-Joseph-Pelletier.

"Pharmaceutical Research by a Commercial House." 1906. *American Druggist and Pharmaceutical Record.* https:// books.google.com/books.

"The Powers-Weightman-Rosengarten Company." 1925. *Industrial and Engineering Chemistry.* 17(1): 99–100. https://doi.org/10.1021/ie50181a050.

"Prescription Drug Labeling Resources." 2020. U.S. Food and Drug Administration. https://www.fda.gov/drugs/ laws-acts-and-rules/prescription-drug-labeling-resources.

"Prescription Drug Monitoring Programs (PDMPs)." 2020. Centers for Disease Control and Prevention. https://www .cdc.gov/drugoverdose/pdmp/providers.html.

"Public Law 215. Chapter 578." 1951. Govinfo. https://www .govinfo.gov/content/pkg/STATUTE-65/pdf/STATUTE-65-Pg648.pdf.

Régnier, Christian. 2020. "A Touch of France: The Medical Faculty of Montpellier: One Thousand Years of Medicine." Medicographia. https://www.medicographia.com/2015/10/ the-medical-faculty-of-montpellier-one-thousand-years-of-medicine/.

Reilly, Gregory W. 2006. "The FDA and Plan B: The Legislative History of the Durham-Humphrey Amendments and the Consideration of Social Harms in the Rx-OTC Switch." Harvard Law School. https://dash .harvard.edu/bitstream/handle/1/8965550/Reilly06.pdf.

"The Rise of Orphan Drugs." 2019. AHIP (America's Health Insurance Plans). https://www.ahip.org/wp-content/ uploads/IB_OrphanDrugs-1004.pdf.

Sasich, Larry D. 2000. "Comments on the Prescription Drug Marketing Act of 1987." Public Citizen. https://www .citizen.org/article/comments-on-the-prescription-drug-marketing-act-of-1987.

Secon, Holly. 2020. "The US Death Rate from the Coronavirus Is 49 Times Higher than the Flu. See How They Compare by Age Bracket." *Business Insider.* https://www.businessinsider.com.au/ coronavirus-death-rate-us-compared-to-flu-by-age-2020-6.

"Semi-Synthetic Opioids." n.d. Drugbank. https://www .drugbank.ca/categories/DBCAT003866.

Seoane-Vazquez, Enrique, et al. 2008. "Incentives for Orphan Drug Research and Development in the United States." *Orphanet Journal of Rare Diseases.* 3: 33. doi: 10.1186/1750-1172-3-33.

Sertürner, F. W. 1817. "Über das Morphium, eine Neue Salzfähige Grundlage, und die Mekonsäure, als Hauptbestandteile des Opiums." *Annalen der Physik.* 25: 56–90.

Sigerist, Henry E. 1941. "Laudanum in the Works of Paracelsus." *Bulletin of the History of Medicine.* 9(5): 530–544.

Sinha, Jay. 2001. "The History and Development of the Leading International Drug Control Conventions." Ottawa: Library of Parliament. https://sencanada.ca/ content/sen/committee/371/ille/library/history-e .htm#A.%20The%201909%20Shanghai%20Conference.

Small, Lyndon F. 1932. "Chemistry of the Opium Alkaloids: Thebaine." https://books.google.com/books/about/ Chemistry_of_the_Opium_Alkaloids.html.

Suvarna, Viraj. 2010. "Phase IV of Drug Development." *Perspectives in Clinical Research.* 1(2): 57–60. https://www .ncbi.nlm.nih.gov/pmc/articles/PMC3148611/.

"Synthetic Opioids: The Ugly and Deadly Truth." 2020. Northpoint Washington. https://www.northpoint washington.com/blog/synthetic-opioids-ugly-deadly-truth/.

Takebe, Tohru, Ryoka Imai, and Shunsuke Ono. 2018. "The Current Status of Drug Discovery and Development as Originated in United States Academia: The Influence of Industrial and Academic Collaboration on Drug Discovery and Development." *Clinical and Translational Science*. 11(6): 597–606. doi: 10.1111/cts.12577.

Teall, Emily K. 2014. "Medicine and Doctoring in Ancient Mesopotamia." *Grand Valley Journal of History*. https://scholarworks.gvsu.edu/gvjh/vol3/iss1/2/.

"Telemedicine Prescribing of Controlled Substances: What Is the Ryan Haight Act?" 2017. Foley & Lardner, LLP. https://www.prms.com/media/2330/ryan-haight-act.pdf.

"2019 National Drug Threat Assessment." 2019. Drug Enforcement Administration. https://www.dea.gov/sites/default/files/2020-01/2019-NDTA-final-01-14-2020_Low_Web-DIR-007-20_2019.pdf.

"Unapproved Drugs." [2020]. U.S. National Library of Medicine. https://dailymed.nlm.nih.gov/dailymed/search.cfm.

Wagner, B. B. 2019. "The Ebers Papyrus: Medico-Magical Beliefs and Treatments Revealed in Ancient Egyptian Medical Text." Ancient Origins. https://www.ancient-origins.net/artifacts-ancient-writings/ebers-papyrus-0012333.

"What Is the U.S. Pharmacopeia?" 2015. Quality Matters. https://qualitymatters.usp.org/what-us-pharmacopeia.

Wilson, Stephen. 1942. *Food & Drug Regulation*. Washington, D.C.: American Council on Public Affairs. https://babel.hathitrust.org/cgi/pt.

Wisniak, Jaime. 2013. "Pierre-Jean Robiquet." *Educación Química*. 24(Supp 1): 139–149. https://doi.org/10.1016/S0187-893X(13)72507-2.

Wright, C. R. A. 1874. "On the Action of Organic Acids and Their Anhydrides on the Natural Alkaloids. Part I." *Journal of the Chemical Society*. 27: 1031–1043. https://www.thevespiary.org/rhodium/Rhodium/Vespiary/talk/files/4132-On-the-action-of-organic-acids-and-their-anhydrides-on-the-natural-alkalo%C3%AFds.-Part-I6d99.pdf.

Young, James Harvey. 1961/2015. *The Toadstool Millionaires: A Social History of Patent Medicines in America Before Federal Regulation*. Princeton, NJ: Princeton University Press.

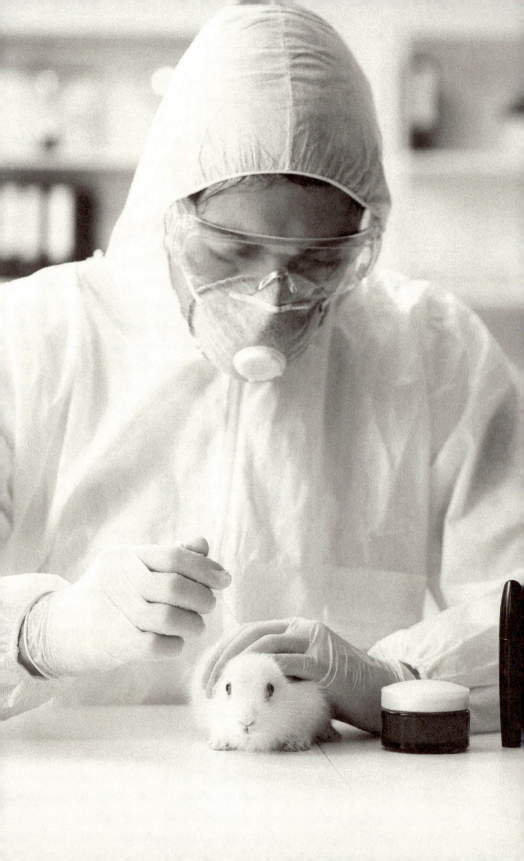

Prescription drugs are a basic and invaluable part of human society today. These products have saved many lives and brought relief to untold numbers of other individuals. However, the discovery, development, and use of prescription drugs have not come about without the advent of a host of new problems and issues. These issues range from the methods for testing new drugs to the possible misuse of prescription drugs, to the economics of drug production and use in the United States and other parts of the world. This chapter explores some of the most common of these problems and issues, along with a consideration of some possible solutions for these dilemmas and controversies.

Testing New Drugs

For as long as humans have searched for new medicines, they have been guided by two general principles. First, a drug has to "work." That is, it has to cure or ameliorate some disease or other disorder. Second, a drug has to be safe. That is, it cannot cause more damage to a human's health, including causing death, than resolving the condition for which it was invented.

Animal Experimentation

Drug research, from the earliest of days, has adopted two methods to achieve these goals. They involve experimentation with

A scientist conducts an experiment in a lab with a rabbit. (Elnur/Dreamstime.com)

humans and with other living organisms. These principles and approaches are reflected in the procedure used today by the Food and Drug Administration (FDA) for the approval of new drugs. At each step in the process—preclinical testing; clinical testing stages 1, 2, and 3; and posttesting—researchers look for possible harmful effects that will exclude a substance for consideration as a new drug. Along the way, testing is carried out in its earliest stages on animals, ranging from fruit flies to mice and rats, to chimpanzees and dogs. According to the most recent data available, a total of 780,070 classified animals were used in medical experiments in 2018. Of these, the most widely used animal was the guinea pig (171,406 cases), followed by the rabbit (133,364) and the hamster (80,579). These data do not include at least two species that are by far the most popular in medical research, mice and rats, as well as other popular subjects, including most fish, reptiles, birds, and most classes of farm animals ("Research Facility Annual Summary & Archive Reports" 2020). No official counts of these animals exist, but some estimates suggest up to 100 million rats and mice alone are killed each year in the United States in the process of medical testing ("Mice and Rats in Laboratories" 2020).

The dissection of animals dates to at least the fifth century BCE in Greece. The Greek natural philosopher Alcmaeon of Croton is credited with being the first person to practice dissection and, perhaps, vivisection, in about 450 BCE. In a search for the seat of human intelligence, he discovered the optic nerve that carries visual impulses from the eyes to the brain. Similar experiments were conducted on animals by renowned physicians such as Aristotle and Erasistratus. Very little remains of details of these experiments. Aristotle alludes to such research in his two books on animals: *The History of Animals* and *Parts of Animals*. In these books, he laid out a general scheme for the study of living organisms, a scheme in which dissection played an essential role because it allowed the investigator to look directly at the parts of which animals bodies are made and how those parts are connected to each other. The two books also contain a vast amount of information on animal anatomy that Aristotle probably could have obtained only through the dissection of living and dead animals. The books apparently contained drawings at one time (references to the drawings exist in the remaining tests), although the drawings themselves are now lost (Lennox 2011).

This line of research was continued and significantly extended by the great Greek physician Galen (129–ca. 216 CE). Galen regarded the study of dead and living animals by dissection and vivisection as one of the best clues to the anatomy and physiology of human bodies. His research in this area was largely responsible—sometimes with erroneous conclusions—for his overall theory of human health and medicine, which was eventually to dominate medical thought for well over a thousand years. It is for this reason that Galen today is referred to as the father of vivisection (Conner 2017, Guerrini 2003; for more details on this topic, see Franco 2013, Newton 2013, Chapter 1).

The debate over the use of animals in experimental research has raged throughout most of the modern era. On the one hand, some individuals have argued that animals are living creatures worthy of all or most of the same rights attributed to humans themselves. Because we would not consider any research that involves cutting humans open just to learn more about some experimental question moral or ethical, we should not consider performing similar types of research on rats, mice, dogs, cats, chimpanzees, or every fruit flies. On the other sides of the debate, the argument has been that animal experimentation has resulted in enormous benefits to medical science, leading to the discovery of medicines (such as drugs) and techniques that have saved untold numbers of human lives and greatly improved the quality of millions more. For more detailed discussions of this issue, see Garrett (2012) and Newton (2013).

Many countries have taken a position on the use of animals in research experiments. In a few cases, those laws date back more than a hundred years, with legislation gradually evolving with regard to specificity and detail of animals involved. In the United States, the key piece of legislation is the Animal Welfare

Act of 1966 (Public Law 89-544). That Act has been amended eight times to deal with more specific issues relating to the use of animals in research, exhibition, and other settings ("Animal Welfare Act" n.d., "Animal Welfare Act Timeline" n.d.). The adoption of this legislation, however, has not resulted in an end of the debate on the topic, which continues with considerable fervor today. One of the talking points of opponents of animal testing is the increasing availability of alternatives to such research, especially methods that can be used *in vitro*, rather than *in vivo*. See, for example, "Should Animals Be Used for Scientific or Commercial Testing?" (2020).

Human Experimentation

Experiments on humans, both living and dead, has a history somewhat less ancient than that of animal experimentation. That history is, for perhaps obvious reasons, surrounded by far more controversy than is animal experimentation. One might argue that it is more acceptable to cut open a living dog to inspect its biological components than to conduct such an experiment on a living (or even dead) human. Nonetheless, records of greater or lesser validity about human experimentation date as far back as least the third century BCE. Some of the most reliable evidence for such research comes from the work of a school of natural philosophers working in Alexandria during this early period. Perhaps best known of these men are the physicians Herophilus and Erasistratus. Both believed that vivisection and dissection were the best ways to discover how the human body is constructed and how it works. Herophilus was perhaps the more productive of these researchers. According to one scholar, he dissected "the ventricles, choroid plexus, venous sinuses, arachnoid, cranial nerves and their foramina, and many other neuroanatomical structures." He also "named certain structures of the brain based on their shape, for example, the cerebrum (encephalon), cerebellum (parencephalon), torcular herophili, calamus scriptorius, and choroid plexus. He described the bones forming the skull, the intervening sutures, and the membranous coverings of the brain" (Elhadi, et al. 2012, 7).

The work of Herophilus and his colleagues along these lines was apparently made possible by the actions of two pharaohs, Ptolemy I and Ptolemy II, who made available to the researchers about 600 live prisoners who had been condemned to death. Standards of pain and suffering in the pursuit of medical knowledge were lower in these circumstances than they were for other individuals in other cultures (Elhadi, et al. 2012).

Indeed, human history is replete with examples of the use of humans, both living and dead, for medical research. Almost without exception, the subjects of such research have been individuals with little or no say as to their participation in such research: prisoners, condemned felons, members of the military, slaves, hospital patients, children, and the poor and/ or disenfranchised. Space does not permit a detailed review of this history, although some good discussions of the practice are available (see, for example, Goliszek 2011, Sharav 2010). Perhaps the best known and most frequently commented upon of all such studies in the United States is the notorious Tuskegee study of 1932 through 1972. The study was a joint project of the U.S. Public Health Service and the Tuskegee Institute, an institute created in 1881 by black educator Booker T. Washington as a teacher college for black students. The purpose of the study was to record the natural history of syphilis, then a common and serious disease among the black population of the United States.

The study was conducted with 600 black men in the Tuskegee area, 399 of whom had already been infected with syphilis and 201 of whom had not yet been infected. The subjects were not informed of the true nature of the research and told only that it involved a condition known as "bad blood." That term actually covered a variety of ailments among the experimental population, including anemia and fatigue, along with syphilis. Although the study was originally designed to run for six months, it continued for forty years, until its true purpose and poorly designed structure were revealed in a series of news articles in the general press. Among the many criticisms of the experiment, perhaps the most serious was that although penicillin had become available to treat the disease in 1945, the drug was not made available to the subjects of the experiment, both those who were infected and those who were not. As a result, many men who might otherwise have been cured of the disease and saved from death were never offered treatment for the condition. (For a good review of the Tuskegee story, see Reverby 2009).

The many improperly designed and conducted and unethical studies on humans over the years, such as the Tuskegee study, prompted governmental agencies to develop an ever-evolving and improving system for monitoring this type of research. In the United States, for example, the Center for Drug Evaluation and Research of the FDA has created a detailed procedure for the selection of humans for participation in the clinical trials that lead to the approval of a new prescription drug. That procedure consists of two primary elements: informed consent and institutional review boards (IRBs). Informed consent is a key component of any experimental research involving humans today. One formal definition of the term is "the process in which a health care provider educates a patient about the risks, benefits, and alternatives of a given procedure or intervention" (Shah, et al. 2020). That is, a potential participant in a medical experiment must be told exactly what is going to take place in that experiment, what the possible benefits of the research might be, what risks a participant faces, and what alternatives to the procedure are available. Informed consent is not only a moral responsibility of a research team but also mandated by legal requirements of the U.S. Code of Federal Regulations (21 CFR 50.25).

The other element providing protection for participants in clinical trials is the existence of IRBs. IRBs are required for all government-funded research in the United States. Legislation laying out the philosophy and function of such entities is provided in the U.S. Code of Federal Regulations at 45 CFR 46. Every institution in which government-funded research on humans is conducted, such as hospitals, medical schools, other universities and colleges, local or state health organization, or an independent agency, must establish an IRB. That group is responsible for reviewing all research programs designed by a member of the institution, making necessary amendments and other changes, and then approving or disapproving the conduct of the research ("Institutional Review Boards: Frequently Asked Questions" 1998/2019).

Testing Biases

The FDA uses a system of clinical trials to determine whether a candidate molecule can be approved as a safe and efficacious drug. Substances that pass that test then become part of formularies from which prescriptions are written for patients needing treatment for some specific type of disease or disorder. The key point about this system is that drug approval and prescription practices that follow do not usually take into consideration a patient's sex, race, ethnicity, age, or other characteristic. A person diagnosed with liver cancer is likely, for example, to be treated with a drug such as bevacizumab (Avastin). A prescriber may not take into consideration whether the patient is a man or a woman, a Latino or an African American, an individual aged twenty-five or aged seventy, or someone from an Italian or a Chinese background. The drug decision is likely to focus on the disease, not the purpose. Many exceptions, however, exist to that general statement today.

Ever since the date on which clinical trials became part of the drug approval system, questions have arisen as to how, if at all, a person's age, sex, race, ethnicity, or other person characteristic can or should affect her or his participation in a clinical trial. Should, for example, women be banned from taking part in clinical trials for a new drug for the treatment of liver cancer? Should individuals over the age of fifty be excluded? Should special efforts be made to ensure that adequate numbers of African Americans are included in a study?

These questions have been (or not been) at the forefront of discussions about and the conduct of clinical trials for at least five decades. Professional and governmental agencies have taken more or less action on ensuring an equitable distribution of trial participants over this time. For example, the FDA issued a set of guidelines for the conduct of clinical trials in 1977. Those guidelines specifically recommended that women of childbearing age be excluded from Phase I trials of new drugs. This decision was based, to a large extent, on the disastrous results associated with the use of the cancer drug thalidomide in the late 1950s and early 1960s ("Thalidomide" 2019). Almost certainly, an overriding determinant in decisions to exclude women was based on the notion that the biological makeup of the two sexes was sufficiently similar that new medicines would probably have essentially the same effect on both sexes. And since women were the weaker, more vulnerable sex, it was probably better that they be excluded from clinical trials unless some important factor was to change that policy (Liu and Mager 2016, McCarthy 1994, Merkatz 1998).

A somewhat similar analysis led to the exclusion of men and women of different races and ethnic groups. Until relatively recently, it was not clear whether differences among such groups could have any significant effect on their responses to new drugs and other types of medication. In addition, an unpleasant history of the use of African Americans (the Tuskegee study) and other minorities in clinical research probably led to a policy of avoidance of clinical trials among such groups (Barrell 2019).

Yet another group of individuals poorly represented in clinical trials is the aged. This fact is somewhat ironic since older adults make up a large fraction of users of many of the prescription drugs approved and prescribed in the United States. One review team found that individuals over the age of sixty-five make up about two thirds of patients with cancer but constitute less than a quarter of those enrolled in phase II and phase III clinical trials on cancer drugs. The team also found similar patterns of inequality in representation for research on Alzheimer's disease, arthritis, epilepsy, incontinence, and cardiovascular disease. It concluded that such disparities "may limit generalizability, provide insufficient data about positive or negative effects of treatment among specific populations, and hinder much-needed access to new treatments" (Herrera, et al. 2010; also see Rochon, Berger, and Gordon 1998). An important recent analysis of this problem found a somewhat more complex pattern. During the development of fifty-nine new drugs approved for use by the FDA in 2018, only 15 percent of participants in clinical trials were over the age of sixty-five. But a dramatic difference existed among the type of trials conducted, with older adults making up half of the participants in trials on oncology drugs, 11 percent on trials of drugs for infectious diseases, and 3 percent on trials for neurological medications (Scott 2019).

A lower-than-expected participation rate in drug trials for individuals with lower income has also been observed for many years. Hard data for this trend has been difficult to obtain until only recently, but some obvious factors are apparent. For example, participants often have to travel considerable distances to get to a trial site. Also, lower-income individuals may find it less convenient to leave their place of work in order to participate in a trial. In addition, poor people may have less access to social media and the Internet, making them less aware of the opportunity to participate in trials. In any case, the evidence is fairly clear that income is a factor in determining participation in clinical trials. One frequently referenced study (Unger, et al. 2013), for example, found that the fraction of participants in cancer trials was proportional to their income level, with those having an annual income of less than $50,000 being 29 percent less likely to take part in such trials than those with an income of more than $50,000. For a review of and commentary about such studies, see Unger, et al. 2016.

Several researchers have attempted to quantify the sex, race, ethnicity, economic status, age, or other factor(s) involved in the disparity of participation in drug trials. One of the key findings of this research is that the results obtained depend on at least two overriding factors: the type of drug being tested and the population characteristic (such as sex or age) being considered. An important source of these data is an annual publication of the FDA, "Drug Trials Snapshots." That document provides a detailed summary of participation in clinical trials for all of the drugs approved in some given year. For the most recent year available (2019), the FDA found that 72 percent of all participants in drug trials in 2018 were white. The same fraction (72 percent) were women. The next largest fraction of participants was Hispanics, who made up 18 percent of all trial participants, followed by 9 percent black or African American and 9 percent Asians. About a third (36 percent) of all participants were over the age of sixty-five ("2019 Drug Trials Snapshots. Summary Report" 2020).

The interesting point about this report is that these numbers varied dramatically depending on the drug being tested. For example, only 21 percent of those who took part in clinical tests for the drug Caplyta, designed for the treatment of schizophrenia, were white, with 75 percent being black or African American. By comparison, 50 percent of the participants in clinical trials for Trikafta, for the treatment of cystic fibrosis, were women, with only 1 percent being black or African American ("2019 Drug Trials Snapshots. Summary Report" 2020; for earlier reports in this series, see https://www.fda.gov/drugs/drug-approvals-and-databases/drug-trials-snapshots).

Perhaps one of the most remarkable findings was that members of a subgroup are not necessarily well represented in drug trials. For example, the occurrence of multiple myeloma is more than twice as great among African Americans in the United States as among whites (14 cases per 100,000 versus 6 cases per 100,000, respectively). Yet African Americans made up only 10 percent of clinical trial participants for one drug for the treatment of the disease (Darzalex), which compares to 76 percent whites; 4 percent of the clinical trial participants for a second drug for the disease (Empliciti), which compares to 84 percent whites; and 3 percent of the clinical trial participants for a third drug (Farydak), which compares to 63 percent whites (Chen and Wong 2018).

Reforming Drug Trial Inequities

For nearly four decades, the FDA, the National Institutes of Health, and other federal and state agencies have been attempting to deal with problems associated with disparities in drug trial populations. One focus of those efforts has been on trying to get the ratio of such populations to reflect those of society in general. For example, if the fraction of blacks and African Americans is currently 13.4 percent, then designers of drug trials should try to have about that fraction of the trial population in that range. Of course, exceptions to that rule exist. For example, it may not be necessary to include any males in tests of drugs for breast cancer or females in tests of drugs for prostate cancer. The other goal of reform efforts is to have clinical trials designed so that they provide new information about the nature of certain diseases and disorders for which drugs are being tested for specific subgroups. For example, in tests on a new drug for liver cancer, it might be desirable to see how women, blacks and African Americans, Latinos, individuals over the age of sixty-five, and other subgroups might respond to that drug. Then, if and when the drug is approved, that information can be used to more effectively and safely prescribe the drug for those subgroups.

Perhaps the earliest of the FDA documents of this type is the "Guideline for the Format and Content of the Nonclinical Pharmacology/Toxicology Section of an Application" (1987). This document did not deal with human clinical trials but with preclinical tests using animals. It required that researchers ensure that appropriate (usually equal) numbers of male and female animals be used in such tests. At about the same time, the FDA began to recommend that clinical trials analyze drug effects on specific groups, such as older adults, children, sex, race, and those with the medical condition for which the drug is being tested ("Regulations, Guidance, and Reports related to Women's Health" 2019).

An important breakthrough in this history occurred in 1993, when the FDA issued the document FDA Guidance Study and Evaluation of Gender Differences in the Clinical Evaluation of Drugs (U.S. Food and Drug Administration 1993). In that document, the FDA acknowledged the fact that men and women often respond differently to drugs and other types of medical treatments. They also recognized the fact that the 1977 document banning women of childbearing age had resulted in a loss of information as to how these women, and perhaps women of other age groups, might respond to drugs being tested. The document noted that "over the past decade there has been growing concern that the drug development process does not produce adequate information about the effects of drugs in women" ("Study and Evaluation of Gender Differences in the Clinical Evaluation of Drugs" 2020, 1). The document then provided examples in which such deficiencies have occurred in studies of cardiovascular disease, the effects of aspirin, and anti-anginal drugs (Mayo Clinic 2019).

Efforts to include members of other subgroups, such as racial and ethnic groups, were also included in the 1993 legislation described previously. For example, the 1993 directive requiring equal representation of women in clinical trials established the same standard for minorities. That enabling legislation, the NIH Revitalization Act of 1993 (Public Law 103-43), noted, "In conducting or supporting clinical research for purposes of this title, the Director of NIH shall, subject to subsection (b), ensure that . . . women are included as subjects in each project of such research; and . . . (B) members of minority groups are included as subjects in such research." That pattern of including minority groups continued throughout the Act:

> The Director of NIH . . . shall conduct or support outreach programs for the recruitment of women and members of minority groups as subjects in projects of clinical research. ("NIH Policy and Guidelines on the Inclusion of Women and Minorities as Subjects in Clinical Research" 2017; see also https://www.govinfo.gov/content/pkg/BILLS-103s1enr/pdf/BILLS-103s1enr.pdf)

Correcting inequities among people of differing sex, gender, race, ethnicity, and other traits has been an issue of constant concern to the FDA, NIH, and other test-monitoring agencies in the federal and state governments. The following list includes some of the most important of these efforts. This list does not include documents discussed in the narrative previously. URLs listed provide links to the original documents.

1985   New Drug Application (21 CFR 314.50 (d)(5)(v)). For the first time, the FDA requires that researchers collect data on the effects of a drug on special categories of individuals, the very young, older adults, and those with the related disease, and renal failure. (https://www.accessdata.fda.gov/scripts/cdrh/cfdocs/cfcfr/CFRSearch.cfm)

1988   Guideline for the Format and Content of the Clinical and Statistical Sections of an Application. Researchers are advised to provide detailed information about research results "in the major subsets (age, sex, race)." (https://www.fda.gov/media/71436/download)

1989   Guideline for the Study of Drugs Likely to Be Used in the Elderly. This document points out that the action of a new drug is likely to differ significantly for individuals of different ages because of body differences in addition to age itself. It suggests data on these factors be considered and reported. (https://www.fda.gov/media/71114/download)

1992   In response to a congressional inquiry, the General Accounting Office reports that the ratio of women used in clinical drug trials is significantly less than the ratio in the population as a whole. It analyzes the reasons for this discrepancy and suggests actions to correct the situation. (https://www.gao.gov/assets/220/216966.pdf)

1994   The Office of Women's Health is created within the FDA. One of the agency's primary responsibilities is to "[monitor] the inclusion of women in clinical trials and the implementation of guidelines concerning the representation of women in clinical trials and the completion of gender analysis." (https://invivo.pharmaintelligence.informa.com/PS024859/FDA-Office-of-Womens-Health)

1998   The Demographic Rule. This rule is contained within amendments made to the New Drug Application procedure by the FDA. It requires that safety and efficacy data be reported for specific subgroups according to gender, age, and race. (https://www.accessdata.fda.gov/scripts/cdrh/cfdocs/cfcfr/CFRSearch.cfm)

2001   One of the first studies of the use of women in clinical drug trials found that adequate numbers of women were included in all trials between 1998 and 2000 that were studied. It found, however, that reports on drug trials typically failed to include data on the safety and efficacy of drugs on women, compared to men, and that the conditions outlined in the preceding document were largely not being met. (https://www.gao.gov/new.items/d01754.pdf)

2013   The FDA conducted a comprehensive review of all drugs and medical devices approved in 2011 to determine the extent to which they met existing requirements and recommendations for inclusion on the basis of sex, gender, age, race, and ethnicity in clinical trials. The report found that the sex and age distribution in clinical trials corresponded to that of the general population, although that was not true for racial groups. Insufficient data for ethnic groups were available for meaningful analysis. The presentation of drug effects on various subgroups was adequate in some cases for sex and age but not in others and almost never adequate for racial subgroups. (https://www.fda .gov/media/86561/download)

2016   The Office of Women's Health joined with the NIH Office on Research in Women's Health to create the Diverse Women in Clinical Trials Initiative. The program acknowledged that adequate numbers of women were currently enrolled in clinical trials but that greater diversity, in terms of age, race, and ethnicity, was needed for such trials. (https://www.fda.gov/consumers/womens-health-topics/ diverse-women-clinical-trials-campaign-partners)

In conclusion, as of late 2020, it would appear that the ratio of women in clinical trials for new drugs has probably reached the ratio of women in the population as a whole. That statement is not necessarily true for many trials of specific drugs, however. Equity of participants on the basis of age, race, ethnicity, gender, and other traits, however, has apparently not reached that level and is a goal to which researchers should continue to work. For more on continuing deficiencies in this arena, see Franconi, et al. (2019), Hoff (2019), Khan, et al. (2020), Nazha, et al. (2019), Nowogrodzki (2017), and O'Reilly and Snyder (2020).

Prescription Drug Abuse

The term *prescription drug abuse* refers to a condition in which a person "tak[es] a medication in a manner or dose other than prescribed; tak[es] someone else's prescription, even if for a legitimate medical complaint such as pain; or tak[es] a medication to feel euphoria (i.e., to get high)" ("Misuse of Prescription Drugs Research Report" 2020, 2). Consider a situation, for example, in which a parent in a household begins taking the prescription drug Prozac (fluoxetine) for a problem of mild depression. Prozac is one of the most popular antidepressants on the market today. The family might sit down together to discuss how Prozac can help a person to be less depressed, that is, to "feel better."

Then imagine that a son or daughter in the family begins to suppose, "I think I'd like to try a Prozac pill. I feel just fine now, but I wonder what it would be like to feel even better. I think I'll give it a try tonight when no one else is around."

When that "trial" occurs, the daughter or son is a bit surprised. Yes, indeed, she or he does feel a bit of a high that goes beyond any "good feeling" she or he has ever had before. That feeling leads to another "trial" of taking Prozac, with similar results, then another "trial," and another. Before long the son or daughter begins to find it hard *not* to take a Prozac every few days or every day. At that point, the person has developed a *dependence* on the drug. A drug dependence is a condition in which a person requires ("depends upon") ingesting a drug in order to function normally. The term *dependence* has now been replaced in many cases with the term *substance abuse disorder*.

Drug dependence can take one of two forms: physical or psychological. A person's body may have become so accustomed to the ingestion of a drug that it no longer functions normally without that drug. Some symptoms of physical dependence include high blood pressure, weight loss, or loss of energy. Physical dependence is often accompanied by *withdrawal symptoms*, bodily changes that may include headache, nausea, tightness in the chest, problems with breathing, dizziness, sweating, tingling of the skin, and muscle aches.

In other cases, a person's lifestyle begins to change because of drug ingestion. These psychological symptoms include making sure one has always enough of the drug around, stealing or other uncharacteristic actions in order to obtain the needed drug, taking unusual risks when under the influence of a drug, cutting back on social interactions with other people, and not meeting one's normal obligations and responsibilities at home, school, or work.

Continued use of a drug may lead to another state of dependence, known as *addiction*. The difference between drug dependence and drug addiction is not entirely clear. Addiction occurs when neural changes occur in the brain that create even more severe demands for a drug than are present in dependence. Generally, a person can become dependent on a drug without becoming addicted but never becomes addicted without first being dependent on the drug. The language of drug abuse is a matter of considerable disagreement and has undergone a number of changes in recent years. Part of this problem is that somewhat different definitions are used by psychiatrists, drug researchers, counselors, treatment centers, and other groups involved in drug abuse issues. See, for example, Shea (2019).

Types of Prescription Drugs of Abuse
Stimulants

Experts often list three categories of prescription drugs as likely to be abused: stimulants, depressants, and opioids. As their name suggests, stimulants are drugs that increase the rate of any bodily function, primarily the brain and the central nervous system (CNS). Some of the prescription stimulants most commonly used for nonmedical purposes are dextroamphetamine (Dexedrine), methylphenidate (Ritalin and Concerta), and amphetamines (Adderall, a mixture of amphetamine and dextroamphetamine). Some street names for these drugs are bennies, black beauties, crosses, hearts, jif, LA turnaround, R-ball, skippy, the smart drug, vitamin R, kibbles and bits, speed, truck drivers, and uppers.

These drugs have become increasingly popular over the past two decades for the treatment of attention deficit hyperactivity disorder, primarily for children under the age of eighteen. The fraction of children in the United States receiving prescriptions of one of these drugs increased from 4.2 to 5.1 percent among children of ages six to twelve and from 2.3 to 4.0 percent among children of ages thirteen to eighteen during the period 1996 to 2008 (Lakhan and Kirchgessner 2012). Overall, the net amount of the four most common stimulants used doubled between 2006 and 2016 (Piper, et al. 2016). Stimulants are also used for other medical conditions, including narcolepsy, asthma, and depression that do not respond to other treatments. According to the most recent data available, about one million Americans used stimulants for nonmedical purposes in 2017. Among adolescents, the most popular stimulant misused was Adderall, with 6 percent of high school seniors reporting misuse of the drug during the previous year ("Misuse of Prescription Drugs Research Report" 2020).

Most studies of the nonmedical use of prescription stimulants have focused on college students, who report three main reasons for using these drugs. First, drugs provide the kind of high that drug abusers often seek from their substance of choice. This effect is a result, as in the case of opioids, of increased levels of dopamine in the brain produced by the ingestion of a stimulant. Second, stimulants also improve a person's ability to concentrate on studying over longer periods of time without becoming tired or distracted. One widely acknowledged fact about stimulant use in colleges is that the use of such products increases dramatically at the end of a school term, when many students find it necessary to cram for an examination, which may require staying awake and studying for long periods of time for "overnighters."

The third reason that college students take prescription stimulants is that they believe that the drugs will actually improve their intellectual level, making them "smarter." While the first two results of taking stimulants are at least biologically valid, the third is not: there is very little evidence that taking stimulants has any effect on a person's cognitive abilities (Lakhan and Kirchgessner 2012, Table 1).

As with all medications, some side effects are associated with even the carefully controlled use of prescription stimulants. These effects may include headache, nausea, increased blood pressure, dizziness, dry mouth, decreased appetite, weight loss, nervousness, insomnia, tics, visual problems, and allergic reactions. Most of these problems can be resolved fairly easily by changing dosage, adjusting the medication schedule, or switching to a different stimulant.

More serious side effects are also possible, especially when an individual ingests a quantity of stimulant greater than that normally recommended for medical treatment. Among the side effects that have been observed under such circumstances are hypertension, tachycardia (rapid heartbeat), and other cardiovascular disorders; depression, hallucinations, mania, and other psychotic effects; and sudden death (Brande 2020).

CNS Depressants

The term *depressants* usually refers to subclasses of drugs known as tranquilizers and sedatives. These drugs are more commonly called *CNS depressants* because they act on the body's CNS. Three classes of drugs make up the majority of CNS depressants used medically and nonmedically: barbiturates, benzodiazepines, and sleep medications. Some familiar examples of drugs belonging to each category are the barbiturates mephobarbital (Mebaral) and sodium pentobarbital (Nembutal); the benzodiazepines diazepam (Valium), alprazolam (Xanax), estazolam (ProSom), clonazepam (Klonopin), and lorazepam (Ativan); and the soporifics (sleep medications) zolpidem (Ambien), zaleplon (Sonata), and eszopiclone (Lunesta). More complete lists of the drugs in these categories can be found in "Prescription Sedatives (Tranquilizers, Depressants)" (2016). Some of the street names by which these drugs are known include A-minus, barbs, candy, downers, phennies, reds or red birds, tooies, yellows or yellow jackets, and zombie pills.

As their name suggests, CNS depressants have an effect on animal bodies that is just the reverse of what stimulants have. Rather than increasing the rate of bodily functions, depressants tend to slow the pace at which those functions occur. They achieve this result because, once ingested, they begin to increase the rate of a neurotransmitter known as gamma aminobutyric acid (GABA). In the brain and the CNS, GABA molecules have a tendency to bind to nerve cell receptors and inhibit the flow of nerve messages from one neuron to another neuron. This reduction in nerve transmission also reduces the stimulation of muscles, causing the reduction in bodily activity characteristics of CNS depressants.

CNS depressants have a number of important medical applications, such as reducing stress, tension, and anxiety and preventing convulsions, seizure disorders, and panic attacks. They are also used in treating sleep disorders. A number of trade names of CNS depressants have become familiar terms in everyday life because the drugs are so widely used in dealing with the physical and psychological problems created by the hectic life that many people lead today.

Individuals cite a number of reasons for using CNS depressants for nonmedical reasons. As with all drugs, some people just want to experiment with drugs to see what results they will experience. Others start out using a CNS depressant for a legitimate medical reason but later find that they have become addicted to the drug and have problems giving it up. Still others experience the same symptoms for which CNS depressants are legitimately prescribed—for example, stress and anxiety in everyday life—but decide to try to deal with the problem on their own rather than seeking professional help. As an example, one of the CNS depressants that gained wide popularity among illicit drug users at the beginning of the twenty-first century was gamma hydroxybutyrate (or gamma hydroxybutyric acid), better known as GHB. The drug has very few legitimate medical applications (no legal applications in the United States) but became popular among prescription drug abusers because it helped them overcome social inhibitions, providing them a modest high and sense of euphoria and a feeling of relaxation in social settings (Teter and Guthrie 2001).

The immediate side effects of taking a CNS depressant are those one would expect from someone whose bodily reactions have begun to slow down: slurred speech, shallow breathing, sleepiness, disorientation, and lack of coordination, for example. If too much of a CNS depressant is consumed, one's body functions may slow down to the point where life-maintaining functions begin to fail and coma and/or death may occur. Some experts suggest that benzodiazepine overdose may soon become America's most serious drug problem. A large part of that problem occurs because of the number of deaths occurring as a result of benzodiazepine-opioid combination misuse in the United States ("The Next U.S. Drug Epidemic as of 2019" 2020).

Opioids

Almost certainly, the category of prescription drugs of greatest concern for misuse today is the opioids. As mentioned in Chapter One, the 1910s and 1920s were an active period of research on semi-synthetic opioids, resulting in the discovery of oxycodone (1916), hydrocodone (1920), and hydromorphone (1924). For many experts in the field, the discovery of these drugs was an important breakthrough in pharmacology. It heralded the possibility of a whole new class of analgesics for use in treating otherwise intractable pain with only modest risk of addiction. To some observers, oxycodone was regarded as "the miracle drug of the 1930s" ("Combat Addiction and Become the Man You Were Meant to Be" 2015). Recent research has also indicated that the drug was a critical tool for a variety of uses within the Nazi regime during World War II (Ohler 2015).

The first prescription drug containing oxycodone to be approved by the FDA was RoxyBond, a formulation of oxycodone hydrochloride (1950). The prescribing information for the drug warned of "risks of addiction, abuse, and misuse, which can lead to overdose and death." "Assess patient's risk," the label continued, "before prescribing and monitor regularly for these behaviors and conditions" ("Highlights of Prescribing Information" 2017). Interest in the use of opioids as analgesics has continued to grow in both Europe and the United States well into the twenty-first century. A defining moment in this period was the decision by one pharmaceutical company, Purdue Pharma, to begin an aggressive campaign of promotion for one version of their oxycodone drug, OxyContin. OxyContin is a time-release form of oxycodone whose effectiveness extends to a period of twelve hours, which compares to four hours for typical oxycodone tablets.

Some of the tools used by Purdue to promote sales of Oxy-Contin included aggressive sales pitches by representatives to doctors, payments of various kinds to physicians who prescribed the drug, and diminution of possible health effects from the drugs (Keefe 2017). The last of these was among the most important approaches, given the concerns about possible dependence and addiction to opioids resulting from the use of OxyContin. One of the research studies most commonly cited by Purdue representatives was a letter to the *New England Journal of Medicine* published in 1980 by Jane Porter and Hershel Jick, from the Boston University Medical Center (Porter and Jick 1980, 123). The five-sentence letter concluded with the authors' observation that "despite widespread use of narcotic drugs in hospitals, the development of addiction is rare in medical patients with no history of addiction." In fact, they claimed to have found "only four cases of reasonably well documented addiction in [11,882] patients who had a history of addiction" (Porter and Jick 1980, 123). The company also referred to another early study that found no cases of addiction among more than 10,000 patients who had been treated for severe burns in the United States (Perry and Heidrich 1982). With this evidence in hand, Purdue recommended to its sales representatives that the risk of addiction arising out of the use of narcotics such as OxyContin was "less than one percent"

(Meier 2003, 67, 173); retelling of the role of Purdue Pharma and other pharmaceutical companies has been the subject of many articles and books. See, for example, Meier (2018), Newton (2018), *The Opioid Epidemic: Tracking a Crisis* (2019), and Van Zee (2009).

The enthusiasm for opioid use as analgesics among pharmaceutical companies (among other factors) soon began to have its effects on prescribing practices by the nation's physicians. The number of prescriptions for opioids grew from 215,917,663 in 2006 to a peak of 255,207,954 in 2012. Since that year, the number of opioid prescriptions has dropped off to 168,158,611 in 2018, largely because of efforts to bring the misuse of opioids under control by a variety of means ("U.S. Opioid Prescribing Rate Maps" 2020). At the same time, the number of opioids being used for nonmedical reasons began to increase at a similar rate. The number reached a peak of 2.7 million new users in 2002, before beginning to fall off (along with the number of prescriptions written) to about 1.8 million in 2012. According to one report, however, "the overall pool of people continuing to use nonmedically is very large" (National Academies of Sciences, Engineering, and Medicine, et al. 2017).

A key factor in the growth of nonmedical use of opioids was the appearance of enabling factors, such as pill mills and doctor shopping. According to one definition, a pill mill is "a doctor's office, clinic, or health care facility that routinely conspires in the prescribing and dispensing of controlled substances outside the scope of the prevailing standards of medical practice in the community or violates the laws of [a state] regarding the prescribing or dispensing of controlled prescription drugs" ("Pill Mill Initiative" 2011). One example of pill mills was the discovery in 2018 of two pharmacies in the town of Williamson, West Virginia, that had shipped about 20.8 million opioid pills over a ten-year period. Williamson has a population of about 3,200, which means that residents were apparently using 6,500 opioid pills per person over that time period (Bever 2018). For more stories about the existence and operation of pill mills, use the "Search" button for "pill mills," at Drug Enforcement Administration (2020).

The term *doctor shopping* refers to the practice of a person's "obtaining controlled substances from multiple healthcare practitioners without the prescribers' knowledge of the other prescriptions" ("Doctor Shopping Laws" 2012). The practice enables a person to obtain large quantities of a prescription drug for which the person has no medical use. An individual might decide to go "doctor shopping" for a variety of reasons. The person may already have a prescription for a legitimate use of a drug to which he or she has become addicted. By visiting a variety of physicians, that person may be able to get additional drugs on the expired prescription. Or a person may want to buy a prescription drug for the purpose of resale to someone who is addicted to the drug. Some visible signs of doctor shopping are making a doctor's appointment for no apparent health reason, claiming that a medication has been lost and needs to be replaced by new pills, traveling considerable distances from one's home to have a prescription filled, and showing signs, in general, of anxiety over simply having to have a prescription refilled (Schneberg, et al. 2020).

A variety of tools have been developed to reduce the number of individuals who have access to prescription opioids for nonmedical use. One approach has been to pass legislation at both the federal and the state levels to deal with pill mills and doctor shopping. One of the first states to adopt a pill mill law was Florida. In 2010, the state had the nation's highest rate of diversion of opioids for illegal use. One consequence of that dubious record is that an estimated seven Floridians were dying every day in the state because of this problem (Kennedy-Hendricks, et al. 2016). In 2011, the state legislature adopted a so-called anti–pill mill bill whose provisions included increasing administrative and criminal penalties for doctors and clinics convicted of prescription drug trafficking, establishing new standards for doctors who prescribe narcotic drugs, adding requirements for the registration of such drugs, banning doctors from prescribing certain drugs especially likely to be used for nonmedical purposes, increasing the monitoring of pharmacies and companies that dispense prescription drugs, and improving the system for monitoring prescription drug dispensing ("Florida's Prescription Drug Diversion and Abuse Roadmap 2012–2015" 2012).

All fifty states and the District of Columbia have some type of legislation dealing with doctor shopping. Those laws differ from state to state and can be classified as *general* doctor shopping laws or *specific* doctor shopping laws. General doctor shopping laws tend to adopt language from the federal Uniform Controlled Substances Act or the much older Uniform Narcotic Drug Act (which it supplanted), which restricts the sale and purchase of all and any kinds of drugs. The relevant Delaware law, for example, is based on the former statute and the California law on the latter statute. Other states, such as Rhode Island, have two general doctor shopping laws, one based on each of the two federal statutes ("Doctor Shopping Laws" 2012). General doctor shopping laws tend to use language such as "it is unlawful for any person knowingly or intentionally . . . to acquire or obtain or attempt to acquire or obtain, possession of a controlled substance or prescription drug by misrepresentation, fraud, forgery, deception or subterfuge" ("Title 16, Health and Safety, Food and Drugs" 2017).

Other states have more specific and more rigorous laws that make it clear that they refer specifically to the practice of doctor shopping. These laws generally describe and prohibit the practices used by individuals in doctor shopping, as in the Montana law, which makes it illegal for a person to

> knowingly or purposefully [fail] to disclose to a practitioner, . . . that the person has received the same or a similar dangerous drug or prescription for a dangerous drug from another source within the prior 30 days; or . . . knowingly or purposefully [communicate] false or incomplete information to a practitioner with the intent to procure the

administration of or a prescription for a dangerous drug. (45-9-104. "Fraudulently Obtaining Dangerous Drugs" 2017)

While many public health and law enforcement agencies are generally enthusiastic about the potential for doctor shopping laws as a way of reducing the illegal use of prescription drugs, some legal and civil rights specialists have expressed concerns about the possible intrusion of such laws on an individual's privacy. They argue that a person's medical records should be sacrosanct and that developing databases that can be shared among doctors, pharmacists, law enforcement officers, and others is a substantial threat to anyone's privacy ("ACLU Asks Court to Protect Confidentiality of Rush Limbaugh's Medical Records" 2004, Schwartzapfel 2017).

One of the most popular approaches to the prevention of prescription drug abuse has been the tracking and monitoring of prescription drug sales. This approach is used by individual states rather than by the federal government. It had its origin in the creation of the California Triplicate Prescription Program (TPP) in 1939. In that program, every prescription for Schedule II drugs had to be written in triplicate: one copy went to a central state recording office (the office of the state attorney general), a second copy remained with the prescriber, and a third copy stayed with the dispensing pharmacy. Over time, the California TPP developed more efficient methods of carrying out this program, changing from written prescriptions to electronic transmissions. Also, additional states adopted programs similar to the California TPP, all with a similar philosophy and similar goals but with a variety of details as to how they operate. Today, such programs are called prescription drug monitoring programs (PDMPs). They exist in forty-nine of fifty states and the District of Columbia. As of October 2020, Missouri is the only state without a PDMP ("Making Use of Your State's Prescription Drug Monitoring Program" 2020,

"Policy Changes Could Bolster Prescription Drug Monitoring Programs" 2020).

PDMPs have a number of benefits. Most importantly, they allow governmental agencies ranging from public health offices to law enforcement agencies to keep track of prescriptions that are being written for drugs that have the potential for non-medical use, such as opioids, stimulants, and depressants. They alert these agencies to the possibility that specific prescribers, dispensers, and/or users may be involved in the nonmedical use of these drugs. PDMPs also make possible a variety of educational programs for prospective abusers of prescription drugs as well as for the general public. They also provide the data and statistics on which such educational programs can be based (Alogailia, Ghania, and Shahb 2020).

Although the federal government has no part in the administration, operation, or other activity of state PDMPs, it does provide financial assistance to states for the development and enhancement of those programs. The primary source of funding for this activity is the Harold Rogers Prescription Drug Monitoring Grant Funding Program, named for Representative Harold Rogers (R-KY). Rogers introduced the legislation in 2001 to the U.S. Congress, which was eventually adopted the following year, creating the program that now carries his name. States that receive grants from the program are free to use them for any one of a variety of purposes, such as collecting and using data to determine drug abuse trends in a state, developing and carrying out the evaluation of existing drug prevention programs, contributing to the development of prescription drug abuse prevention programs, and enabling Native American communities to create and operate prescription drug abuse prevention programs and coordinating their efforts with those of the state in which they are located ("Harold Rogers Prescription Drug Monitoring Program" 2010).

One of the most critical questions relating to these programs is the extent to which they make it more difficult for physicians to prescribe opioids for legitimate medical purposes, such as the relief of chronic pain. A doctor may be concerned, for example, that he or she will be prosecuted for prescribing an opioid drug for pain relief in too large doses or too frequently. As a consequence, the doctor may not provide a patient with the pain relief he or she legitimately needs. In one study on this issue, researchers found that the prescription of opioids for pain relief dropped by about 30 percent after the adoption of a PDMP in a state. They concluded that there was no significant impact on the overall prescribing of pain medication, although they were unable to state whether patients' pain was effectively managed under the circumstances (Bao, et al. 2016).

How effective have these and other programs been in dealing with the nation's opioid epidemic? There is probably no simple answer to that question. Some of the most obvious data needed to do so are (1) the number of emergency department visits and hospitalizations for nonfatal cases of drug overdose and (2) the number of deaths attributed to opioid overdose. In both cases, data seem to be trending upward from the late 1990s to the present day. Table 2.1 shows the number of inpatient hospital stays attributed to opioid overdose. Brief, intermittent downward trends exist, but the long-term overall trend appears to be an increase in such events. Trends for deaths from opioid overdose (Table 2.2) appear to be similar for those for hospital stays but with few or no decreases even intermittently.

Table 2.1 Opioid-Related Emergency Department Visits and Hospital Stays per 100,000 Population

Year	Emergency Department Visits	Inpatient Stays (stays per 100,000)
2005	89.1	136.8
2006	91.8	164.2
2007	82.6	159.0
2008	94.1	165.7
2009	107.4	181.4
2010	117.5	198.8*
2011	131.2	208.0*

Year	Emergency Department Visits	Inpatient Stays (stays per 100,000)
2012	146.8	204.9*
2013	166.2	212.1*
2014	177.7	229.2*
2015	n/a	289.0*
2016	n/a	296.7*
2017	n/a	291.5*

*Data for fourth quarter of each year.

Source: "Opioid-Related Hospital Use Rate of Inpatient Stays per 100,000 Population." 2020. HCUP Fast Facts. https://www.hcup-us.ahrq.gov/faststats/OpioidUseServlet. August 30, 2020; Weiss, Audrey J., et al. 2017. "Opioid-Related Inpatient Stays and Emergency Department Visits by State, 2009–2014." HCUP. https://www.hcup-us.ahrq.gov/reports/statbriefs/sb219-Opioid-Hospital-Stays-ED-Visits-by-State.jsp. August 30, 2020.

Table 2.2 Drug Overdose Deaths in the United States, 1999–2018

Year	Total	Male	Female
1999	16,849	11,258	5,591
2000	17,415	11,563	5,852
2001	19,394	12,658	6,736
2002	23,518	15,028	8,490
2003	25,785	16,399	9,386
2004	27,424	17,120	10,304
2005	29,813	18,724	11,089
2006	34,425	21,893	12,532
2007	36,010	22,298	13,712
2008	36,450	22,468	13,982
2009	37,004	22,593	14,411
2010	38,329	23,006	15,323
2011	41,340	24,988	16,352
2012	41,502	25,112	16,390
2013	43,982	26,799	17,183
2014	47,055	28,812	18,243
2015	52,404	32,957	19,447
2016	63,632	41,558	22,074
2017	70,237	46,552	23,685
2018	67,367	44,941	22,426

Source: "Data Brief 356. Drug Overdose Deaths in the United States, 1999–2018." 2020. National Center for Health Statistics. https://www.cdc.gov/nchs/data/databriefs/db356_tables-508.pdf#page=1. August 29, 2020. Data for Figure 1 in report.

Table 2.3 Drug Overdose Deaths in the United States, 1999–2018, by Opioid Type

Year	Any Opioid	Heroin	Natural and Semi-Synthetic Opioids	Methadone	Synthetic Opioids Other than Methadone
1999	8,050	1,960	2,749	784	730
2000	8,407	1,842	2,917	986	782
2001	9,496	1,779	3,479	1,456	957
2002	11,920	2,089	4,416	2,358	1,295
2003	12,940	2,080	4,867	2,972	1,400
2004	13,756	1,878	5,231	3,845	1,664
2005	14,918	2,009	5,774	4,460	1,742
2006	17,545	2,088	7,017	5,406	2,707
2007	18,516	2,399	8,158	5,518	2,213
2008	19,582	3,041	9,119	4,924	2,306
2009	20,422	3,278	9,735	4,696	2,946
2010	21,089	3,036	10,943	4,577	3,007
2011	22,784	4,397	11,693	4,418	2,666
2012	23,166	5,925	11,140	3,932	2,628
2013	25,052	8,257	11,346	3,591	3,105
2014	28,647	10,574	12,159	3,400	5,544
2015	33,091	12,989	12,727	3,301	9,580
2016	42,249	15,469	14,487	3,373	19,413
2017	47,600	15,482	14,495	3,194	28,466
2018	46,802	14,996	12,552	3,023	31,335

Source: "Data Brief 356. Drug Overdose Deaths in the United States, 1999–2018." 2020. National Center for Health Statistics. https://www.cdc.gov/nchs/data/databriefs/db356_tables-508.pdf#page=1. August 29, 2020. Data for Figure 3 in report.

Shown are raw data.

Perhaps of equal interest is in the qualitative aspects of these trends, in comparison to the quantitative aspects. Some experts point out that the so-called opioid epidemic actually consists of three somewhat different "waves." The first wave began in the 1990s, with nonmedical use of prescription opioids accounting for the greatest number of deaths. A second wave appeared in about 2010, with many users shifting their drug of choice to heroin. The third and most recent wave can be dated to about 2013, when the drug of choice became fentanyl (Kunzmann

Table 2.4 Drug Overdose Deaths in the United States, 1999–2018, by Opioid Type

Year	Any Opioid	Heroin	Natural and Semi-Synthetic Opioids	Methadone	Synthetic Opioids Other than Methadone
1999	2.9	0.7	1.0	0.3	0.3
2000	3.0	0.7	1.0	0.4	0.3
2001	3.3	0.6	1.2	0.5	0.3
2002	4.1	0.7	1.5	0.8	0.4
2003	4.5	0.7	1.7	1.0	0.5
2004	4.7	0.6	1.8	1.3	0.6
2005	5.1	0.7	1.9	1.5	0.6
2006	5.9	0.7	2.3	1.8	0.9
2007	6.1	0.8	2.7	1.8	0.7
2008	6.4	1.0	3.0	1.6	0.8
2009	6.6	1.1	3.1	1.5	1.0
2010	6.8	1.0	3.5	1.5	1.0
2011	7.3	1.4	3.7	1.4	0.8
2012	7.4	1.9	3.5	1.2	0.8
2013	7.9	2.7	3.5	1.1	1.0
2014	9.0	3.4	3.8	1.1	1.8
2015	10.4	4.1	3.9	1.0	3.1
2016	13.3	4.9	4.4	1.0	6.2
2017	14.9	4.9	4.4	1.0	9.0
2018	14.6	4.7	3.8	0.9	9.9

Source: "Data Brief 356. Drug Overdose Deaths in the United States, 1999–2018." 2020. National Center for Health Statistics. https://www.cdc.gov/nchs/data/databriefs/db356_tables-508.pdf#page=1. August 29, 2020. Data for Figure 3 in report.

Shown are deaths per 100,000.

and Walter 2020). Fentanyl is a synthetic opioid analgesic listed as a Schedule II drug. It is approved for use in the treatment of severe pain, especially in postsurgical settings. It has a potency fifty to one hundred times greater than that of morphine, which it often replaces in therapeutic settings ("Fentanyl Drug Facts" 2019).

The slight dip in opioid overdose hospitalizations and deaths in 2018 prompted some observers to hope that there had finally been a turnaround in the opioid epidemic in the United

States. But it turned out not to be the case. In its most recent annual report on drug overdose deaths, the National Center on Health Statistics (NCHS) found that the number of deaths from opioid overdose rose from 67, 367 in 2018 to 70,630 in 2019 (the most recent year for which data are available) ("Data Brief 394" 2020).

One factor that may have contributed to the continued spread of opioid overdose deaths was the rise of the COVID-19 pandemic in 2020. Several reasons have been suggested for this connection. First, the presence of the new pandemic may well have taken over news space in periodicals and the Internet, moving opioid issues to the back burner of the news cycle. Other possible connections are stay-at-home orders, which may have reduced the availability of treatment programs for opioid abusers, and social isolation policies, which may have caused certain behavioral changes that may have led to increased use of opioids (Keenan 2020). One piece of evidence for the connection between opioid misuse and COVID-19 can be found in a study conducted by Millennium Health in July 2020. That study found an increase of 31.96 percent for un-prescribed fentanyl in urine samples studied, along with increases of 19.96 percent for methamphetamine and 12.53 percent for heroin ("Significant Changes in Drug Use During the Pandemic" 2020). Over the same period, a study by the University of Baltimore Center for Drug Policy and Enforcement reported an increase of 17.59 percent in opioid overdose reports for the region (Alter and Yeager 2020). Based on data such as these, it appears that the opioid epidemic has clearly not "gone away" and may not even be decreasing in intensity ("Fatal Drug Overdoses Hit a Record High Last Year" 2020).

The Cost of Prescription Drugs

Health care costs in the United States have been an issue of major importance for at least the past two decades. As far back as 1960, the average annual cost of health care for the typical

American was about $27 per year. Over the next forty years, that number mushroomed to nearly $1,370 per person per year, and two decades later, it had reached $3,649 per person per year (Table 2.5). A similar increase in the share of the national budget spent on health care occurred. In 1960, about 5 percent of the U.S. budget went to health care costs. Today, that number is nearly three times greater, at 17.7 percent of the gross domestic product (GDP).

Table 2.5 Cost of National Health Care, 1960–2018

o	Total Cost[1]	Per Capita Cost ($)	Percentage of Increase[2]	Percentage of GDP
1960	27.2	146	n/a	5.0
1970	74.6	355	10.6	6.9
1980	255.3	1,108	13.1	8.9
1990	721.4	2,843	10.9	12.1
2000	1,369.2	4,855	6.6	13.4
2001	1,486.2	5,218	8.5	14.0
2002	1,628.7	5,666	9.6	14.9
2003	1,767.6	6,097	8.5	15.4
2004	1,895.8	6,479	7.2	15.5
2005	2,023.8	6,854	6.8	15.5
2006	2,156.2	7,232	6.5	15.6
2007	2,294.4	7,624	6.4	15.9
2008	2,397.1	7,890	4.5	16.3
2009	2,491.8	8,131	4.0	17.2
2010	2,593.2	8,394	4.1	17.3
2011	2,682.6	8,625	3.4	17.3
2012	2,791.1	8,908	4.0	17.2
2013	2,875.0	9,113	3.0	17.1
2014	3,025.4	9,518	5.2	17.3
2015	3,199.6	9,995	5.8	17.6
2016	3,347.4	10,379	4.6	17.9
2017	3,487.3	10,742	4.2	17.9
2018	3,649.4	11,172	4.6	17.7

Source: National Health Expenditure Data. 2020. Centers for Medicare & Medicaid Services, Table 1. https://www.cms.gov/Research-Statistics-Data-and-Systems/Statistics-Trends-and-Reports/NationalHealthExpendData/NationalHealthAccountsHistorical.

[1] In billions of dollars.
[2] From previous year shown.

The Data

Historically, the United States has spent a larger fraction of its GDP for health care than all other developed countries worldwide. For example, the differential between members of the United States and other members of the Organization for Economic Cooperation and Development in 1980 was about 3 percent. Today, that difference is closer to 8 percent. According to the latest data available, the United States spent about 16.9 percent of its GDP on health care in 2018, compared to the next highest nation, Switzerland, which spent 12.2 percent of its GDP, all the way down to New Zealand, which spent about 9.3 percent of its GDP on health care (Tikkanen and Abrams 2020).

Health care costs consist of several components. According to the most recent data available (2018), that cost distribution consisted of 33 percent hospital care, 20 percent physician and clinical services, 9 percent retail prescription drugs, and 5 percent other products and services. ("National Health Expenditures 2018 Highlights" 2020). Data on all aspects of health care and prescription drug costs vary from source to source and depend on a variety of factors. The term *retail prescription drugs*, for example, refers only to drugs provided through retail outlets, such as independent pharmacies, chain pharmacies, food stores, and mass merchandisers. It does not include drugs dispensed through clinics, hospitals, physicians' offices, or pharmacies within a closed health care system ("Prescription Drug Spending in the U.S. Health Care System" 2018). The true cost of all prescription drugs, then, can be significantly higher than that for retail drugs only. According to one survey of the data, for example, the cost of *all* prescription drugs (retail and nonretail) in 2018 made up 16.8 percent of all health care costs, nearly twice the number quoted previously here ("A Look at Drug Spending in the U.S." 2018).

The long-term trends in prescription drug costs in developed nations over the past half century are similar to those for health care costs overall. In 1980, for example, the nation with the highest per capita costs for prescription drugs was France, which recorded a cost of $86.1 per person per year. Next on the list were the Netherlands, at $59.1 per person per year, and the United States, at $53.0 per person per year. Over time, that pattern of spending changed fairly dramatically. By 1998, the United States had surpassed France as the nation with the highest per capita drug costs, at $320.8 per person per year, compared to $308.1 per person per year in France. That differential continued to grow significantly over the next twenty years. By 2018, the average cost of prescription drugs in the United States was $1,220 per person per year, followed by Switzerland ($963 per person per year), Canada ($832 per person per year), Japan ($838 per person per year), and Germany ($823 per person per year) (Sarnak, Squires, and Bishop 2017, "Pharmaceutical Spending per Capita in Selected Countries as of 2018" 2020).

The issue of soaring prescription drug prices has had its moments of drama over the past few years, moments when the issue received widespread public attention. One such event occurred in 2015, when hedge fund manager Martin Shkreli raised the price of the drug Daraprim (pyrimethamine) by a factor of 56, from $13.50 to $750 per pill essentially overnight. Daraprim had been approved by the FDA in 1953 for use primarily as an antimalarial and an antiparasitic medication. Its patent coverage had expired, and no other competing drug was available on the market. Shkreli took this action primarily because there was no viable competitor drug. He acted largely as part of his plan to make the newly created Turing Pharmaceutical (founded in 2015) a profitable enterprise (Sanneh 2016).

A similar case of rapidly inflated prices involved the use of a product known commercially as the Epi-Pen, an injection device for emergency use in the treatment of allergic reactions. Many individuals, including children and young adults, are required to carry Epi-Pens with them at all times to deal with unexpected allergic reactions. In 2016, Epi-Pen's manufacturer, Mylan, raised the price of a two-pen package in the United States from about $57 to more than $500. (As always, drug prices can vary substantially for a number of reasons.) One reason for the increase, according to an observer, was "because they [Mylan] could" (Willingham 2016). For later developments in this case, see Marsh (2018).

The story of prescription drug price changes for the vast majority of such drugs is very different from that of the two stories outlined previously. For example, the actual price that a consumer pays for a prescription drug can vary widely depending on the insurance plan (if any) he or she may have and the method used by that plan to determine a drug price. A standard method for expressing prescription drug prices in the United States in any one year is the *CPI prescription drug index*, which is roughly comparable to the *consumer price index*, used by the U.S. Bureau of Labor Statistics (BLS) to express the average change in prices over time that consumers pay for a basket of goods and services.

Given those limitations, various organizations attempt to measure and express the change in prescription drug prices from year to year. For example, the website GoodRx reports on changes in prescription drug prices in the United States over certain given time periods on a regular basis. Its January 2020 report found that 639 drugs had increased in price by an average of 6 percent, of which 619 brand drugs had increased by an average of 5.2 percent (Marsh 2020a). Some prices changes for specific drugs are as follows (Marsh 2020a):

Eliquis: 6.0%
Truvada: 4.8%
Armour Thyroid: 5.0%
Vyvanase: 5.0%
Symbicort: 3.0%

Bystolic: 5.0%

Diazepam (generic Vallium): 7.8%

Xarelton: 4.9%

Marplaon: 14.9%

Contempla XR: 13.2%

Neoprofen: 10.0%

Percocet: 9.9%

A more updated addendum to the previously mentioned report, focusing on mid-year drug prices, can be found at Marsh (2020b). These numbers do not mean very much unless they are compared to general changes in cost of living in the United States over the same period of time. The overall BLS CPI for that period of time was 2.5, meaning that prescription drug costs increased by about 140 percent compared to other costs of living ("TED: The Economics Daily" 2020).

So is the current outcry over the increasing cost of prescription drugs justified? That's a tough question to answer. In 2019, The President's Council of Economic Advisors issued a report arguing that whatever recent past history has been, the cost of prescription drugs has actually been dropping in the year preceding the report. Perhaps the report's most influential conclusion is that the CPI-Rx was actually falling from the beginning of 2018 to the date of the report (October 2019). A graphic representation of that trend has now become common in the literature ("Measuring Prescription Drug Prices" 2019, Figure 1, page 3). The report then went on to explain why this conclusion appears to be at variance to the general view that prescription drug prices are increasing at an unacceptable rate. Its authors suggested, for example, that news reports may be focused on a single drug or a small class of drugs. Or an analyst's conclusions may be based on a biased set of drugs rather than a complete record of all drugs available. Or reports of concern may not take into consideration the extent to which various drugs are used, treating them all as equally important in that regard (Taylor 2019).

Causes

So differences of opinion exist about the status and direction of prescription drug prices. The fact remains that a review of the popular and most technical literature is that, as far as individual Americans are concerned, those prices are too high in the country and are likely to continue increasing over the foreseeable future. One important report from the Centers for Medicare and Medicaid in 2020 projected that the total cost of prescription drugs in the United States would rise from $333.4 billion in 2017 to $576.7 billion in 2027, an increase of 73.0 percent. The projected increase in prescription drug prices *per capita* was then estimated to be about 60 percent, from $1,025 per capita in 2017 to $1,635 per capita in 2027 ("Prescription Drug Expenditures" 2020, Table 11). Of the 2027 total, about 13 percent is expected to come from direct out-of-pocket payments by individuals, with the remaining coming from some unknown and unpredictable mix of Medicare, Medicaid, private health insurance, and other third-party payers.

Corporate Expenses and Profits

Substantial amounts of time and energy have been devoted to discovering *why* drug prices in the United States are so high and why they continue to increase at significant rates. The answers to these questions, researchers and policy makers believe, may lead to the development of methods for reducing such costs and increases. So how can the price trends in prescription drug prices be explained? Quite obviously, one major factor in determining a drug's retail price is the cost of developing the drug for FDA approval. Several studies have been conducted on the cost of research and development for any given drug. One such study, focused on the cost of cancer drugs, found the data for the five most expensive products (see Table 2.6).

Table 2.6 Cancer Drugs with Highest Development Costs, 2015

Drug	Maker	R&D Cost
Cabozantinib	Exelisis	1,950.8
Ruxolitinib	Incyte Corporation	1,097.8
Brentuximab	Seattle Genetics	899.2
Eculizamab	Alexion Pharmaceuticals	817.6
Irinotecan	Merrimack Pharmaceuticals	815.8

Source: Prasad and Mailankody (2017, p. 1571).

Costs shown are in millions of dollars.

Another measure of the cost of drug research and development is the total amount a company budgets for this expense. These numbers can be extremely high. One report on the budgets for drug research and development showed the following data for ten large companies:

Roche	11.06
Johnson & Johnson	10.80
Merck	9.75
Novartis	9.074
Pfizer	8.006
Sanof	6.961
Bristol-Myers-Squibb	6.345
Astra/Zeneca	5,932
Eli Lilly	5,307
GlaxoSmithKline	5,196

Source: Taylor (2020).

Shown are 2018 figures in billions of dollars.

Pharmaceutical companies commonly point to the cost of developing new drugs as a major factor for setting (and raising) the price of their products. One company, for example, has explained in their own publications that drug prices are driven to a significant extent to "generate the revenues we need to fund research into future treatments and cures" ("Transforming Lives" 2019, 27). Still, that explanation is not totally satisfactory. Numerous studies have shown that companies typically spend more on advertising and marketing of their products than they do for research and development. One such study, for example, found that "research and development is only about 17 percent of total spending in most large drug companies" (Kodjak 2019); a related study mentioned in this source is Hernandez, et al. (2019).

So the pricing of a new drug depends to at least some extent on the cost of producing the drug and having it approved by the FDA and setting aside enough money for future research and development. How, then, does a company decide, given these data, what a "fair price" for a new drug should be? In almost all countries around the world, the answer to that question is a bit complicated, involving both the specific drug company and the federal agencies. In the United Kingdom, for example, the main buyer for prescription drugs is the nation's National Health Service, the free, comprehensive, and universal health care system adopted in 1948. The price of those drugs is determined in consultation between manufacturers and the UK Department of Health as outlined by the Pharmaceutical Price Regulation Scheme, a voluntary agreement between the federal government and the pharmaceutical industry ("Drug Pricing" 2010). For a detailed description of this process, see Castle, Kelly, and Gathani (2020). An increasingly important element in this system is the principle of *value-based pricing*, that is, the setting of the price of a drug at least partly as a reflection of the value it provides to individual consumers and the general market overall (Claxton, Sculpher, and Carroll 2011).

In the United States, no such system exists. Pharmaceutical companies can essentially establish a price for a new drug (or reprice an existing drug) at whatever level they choose. For example, the public uproar over Martin Shkreli's inflation of the price for the drug Daraprim was not accompanied by any criminal charges; according to U.S. practices, he was allowed to charge whatever he wanted to for the drug and all other drugs in the company's portfolio. Shkreli was, however, convicted of other crimes unrelated to drug price inflation and sentenced to seven years in prison with a $7.36 million fine (Clifford 2018). Generally speaking, then, "U.S. law allows pharmaceutical manufacturers to price their products at whatever level they believe the market will bear and to raise prices over time without limit" (Fralick and Kesselheim 2019, citing Luo, Avorn, and Kesselheim 2015).

For the general public, pharmaceutical company profits are among the most important factors responsible for rising drug costs. In a 2019 poll by the Kaiser Family Foundation, the most frequently expressed reason for drug prices, according to respondents, was profits made by drug companies, with 80 percent of those interviewed giving this answer. The next most common reason for rising drug prices in this poll was costs related to research and development (69 percent of respondents), followed by profits made by prescription drug benefits management companies (63 percent), and costs of marketing and advertising (52 percent). Overall, only 3 percent of respondents believed that drug companies raised drug prices "fairly" "a lot" of the time, with 22 percent selecting the response "somewhat." By far the more common responses were that companies "not at all" or "not too much" raised drug prices "fairly" (43 percent and 31 percent of respondents, respectively) (Kirzinger, et al. 2019).

Concerns about pharmaceutical company profits as a factor in the rising costs of drugs is understandable. Considerable attention has been paid to the financial bottom line for major drug manufacturing companies in recent years. One summary of these data for 2018 found, for example, the following leaders in profit margins among pharmaceutical companies:

Pfizer	4,114
Johnson & Johnson	3,934
Sanofi	2,594
Merck	1,950
Bristol Myers Squibb	1,901
Amgen	1.859
GlaxoSmithKline	1,836
Novartis	1,624
Eli Lilly	1,150
Astra Zeneca	406

Source: Herman (2018).

Data are for third quarter 2018 in millions of dollars. Companies sometimes lose money, too. Over this period, for example, Allergan lost $38 million. The company was later acquired by Abbvie, in 2020.

An even larger part of increasing drug prices can be attributed to the costs of sale and marketing of products, both new and old, by pharmaceutical firms. Johnson & Johnson, among the world's ten largest drug companies, spent more than twice as much in 2014 selling their products ($17.5 billion) as they did in researching and developing those products ($8.2 billion). Similar trends existed for eight of the remaining nine firms, the only exception being Hoffmann-LaRoche, where research and development accounted for just barely more of the company's budget ($9.3 billion) than for sales and marketing ($9.0 billion) (Anderson 2014). For a subsequent assessment of these data, see Brennan (2019).

A key aspect of corporate financing in rising drug prices involves patent law. Under patent law, a pharmaceutical company can apply for the right to be the sole manufacturer of a drug for some given period of time, now, twenty years. During that time, no other company is allowed to manufacture or sell the same drug or one that is similar to it. The purpose of the patent law is to encourage companies to use profits from drug sales for research and development of new drugs to replace another drug, once its patent has expired. Drug companies have, however, found a way to work around even this generous restriction. They make use of a tactic sometimes known as the *patent thicket*. That term refers to the practice of a company's applying multiple times for protection of a single product. Each time a new patent is approved, the period of time over which a company has control of manufacture and sale of the drug becomes longer.

One recent report has highlighted the extent and effects of this practice ("Overpatented" 2018). The study analyzed patent requests and approvals for the twelve best selling prescription drugs in the United States. Among the findings of that study are the following:

- An average of 125 patent applications (a total of 1,498 applications) were submitted for each of the 12 drugs.
- An average of 71 of those applications (a total of 848 applications) were granted.
- The price change for the twelve drugs in question averaged an increase of 68 percent. Only one of the drugs studied showed an actual decrease in price.
- AbbVie, producer of the world's number one selling drug, Humira, had the largest number of applications: 247.
- Roche/Genentech has patents extending back to 1985 that will protect its drug, Herceptin, until 2033.
- One third of the drugs studied have had price increases of more than 100 percent since 2012 (although the composition of the drug has not had substantial changes during that period).

Other Causes

Corporate expenses and profits are by no means the only reason for rising drug prices. Another important factor in this process is the actions of pharmacy benefit managers (PBMs). A PBM is a third-party agency that manages prescription drug benefits for health insurers, Medicare Part D drug plans, large employers, and other entities responsible for prescription drug distribution. Today, there are more than seventy PBMs operating in the United States, the largest of which are CVS Health (Caremark), with 30 percent of the market, Express Scripts (23 percent), Optum Rx (United Health; 23 percent), Humana Pharmacy Solutions (7 percent), Medimpact Healthcare Systems (6 percent), and Prime Therapeutics (6 percent) ("PBM Companies" 2020, "Market Share of the Top 5 Pharmacy Benefit Managers in the U.S. Prescription Market in 2018" 2020).

The role of PBMs in drug pricing is a bit complicated and can be illustrated by the following example. Suppose that a pharmaceutical company decides to charge $100 for a month's supply of a drug. The company normally does not sell the drug directly to the consumer. Instead, an insurer, such as Medicare or a private insurance company, contracts with a PBM to distribute the drug. The PBM, in turn, contracts with individual pharmacies through which the drug is distributed.

A PBM seldom pays the pharmaceutical company the price the company has decided upon, in this case, $100. Instead, the PBM negotiates a reduced price for the drug, partly as an incentive for agreeing to list the drug in the PBM's formulary. (Recall that the formulary lists the drugs that can be distributed to a consumer.) In this example, assume that the negotiated price is $80. In one sense, then, the PBM has already made a $20 profit based on the company's list price of $100.

The PBM then agrees to sell the drug to pharmacies at its negotiated price, $80 in this example. But pharmacies also pay a PBM a fee for handling negotiations for sale and listing of the drug with the drug company and the insurer. Assume that the fee paid is $10. The cost to the consumer, then, is $90, more than she or he would have paid for the discounted price for the drug. The PBM then makes an additional $10 on the drug from the pharmacy fees. In actual practice, these negotiations can—and often are—a good deal more complicated and, more important, are not made available to the general public (Arnold 2018; "New Drug Pricing Analysis Reveals Where PBMs and Pharmacies Make Their Money" 2019).

In addition to the factors discussed previously, other causes may contribute to the increase in drug costs, usually of less importance than those reviewed here. For a detailed discussion of this issue, see Augustine, Madhavan, and Nass (2018, Chapter 3). For example, mergers and acquisitions among drug companies tend to result in an increase in drug prices for the products of one or both companies. In one study, that increase was found to account for about 5 percent in the increase of a company's drug prices (Bonaime and Wang 2020).

Another factor of growing importance in the cost of prescription drugs is personalized medicine and other advances in health care technology. These advances hold enormous potential for improving the care needed by and provided to individuals with specialized medical conditions that often cannot be treated by conventional medicines and medical devices. This development represents a drift away from the "one solution fits all" approach that currently dominates medical practice. As researchers learn more about the specific characteristics of any one individual's biological makeup, the tailoring of drugs to deal with those unique requirements becomes more important.

One example of this trend was the 2019 approval of the drug Zolgensma (onasemnogene abeparvovec-xioi) by the FDA. The drug was approved for use in the treatment of a rare medical condition, spinal muscular atrophy (SMA), which affects fewer than 25,000 individuals in the United States each year. The cost set for one treatment of the drug by its developer, Novartis, was $2,125,000. The company argued that the cost of keeping SMA patients alive was far in excess of that cost and, therefore, the price was justified (Luxner 2019). According to a recent study, there are at least 300 specialized drugs that fall into the same category as Zolgensma. That is, they are drugs that successfully treat relatively rare medical conditions and often are life-saving medications, but they are also factors contributing to the overall increase in drug prices in the United States ("Medicines in Development for Cell Therapy and Gene Therapy" 2018).

Possible Solutions

Many possible solutions have been suggested for the problem of rising drug prices. Relatively few of these solutions have been successfully implemented. One critical reason for that fact—it should be noted at the outset—relates to the economic system dominant in the United States: capitalism. Capitalism is a system in which private individuals and organizations own capital goods. It is a market economy, in which the production of goods and services is determined by supply and demand. The primary purpose of operating a company in the capitalist system is to make a profit, the so-called *profit motive*. Many companies are conscious of and work toward the alleviation of social ills and problems. But those efforts are not the primary driver of the company's activities. Today, the vast majority of Americans accept the economic philosophy described here and are doubtful about or actively opposed to alternative systems, such as socialism (Newport 2020). Discussions of economic systems are highly complex and are beyond the scope of this text.

So what does this discussion about economic systems have to do with the rise in drug prices? In the simplest possible terms, it explains why pharmaceutical companies usually feel justified in raising drug prices, even when there are no research, development, production, demand, or other reasons for making changes in price structures. The companies' purpose is to make a profit so that they can pay stockholders a reasonable return on their investment and their management a fair salary. The five highest-paid drug company CEOs in 2019 received $58.6 million, $27.1 million, $27.0 million, $26.5 million, and $26.0 million. The pay gap between CEO and average employee wage is 315:1, 293:1, 268:1, 244:1, and 243:1 (Dunn and Pagliarulo 2019).

In simple terms, pharmaceutical companies (like all companies in a capitalist economy) are designed to make profits, so raising drug prices is a legitimate and rational way of doing business. One of the most famous direct commentaries on this point came from Martin Shkreli, whose actions in raising drug prices were described previously. When asked about his decision to raise the price of Daraprim by more than 4,000 percent, Shkreli said, "It's a great business decision that also benefits all of our stakeholders." "There's no doubt," he went on, "I'm a capitalist. . . . I'm trying to create a big drug company, a successful drug company, a profitable drug company. We're trying to flourish." As one of his interviewers then observed, "So there you have it. The unvarnished truth. It was a business decision. It was about money. And screw you" (Miller 2015).

Although somewhat crass, Shkreli's comments probably reflect the thinking of at least some—if not the majority—of pharmaceutical companies. After all, in a capitalist society, do consumers have the right to object if a baker raises his prices on bread by 5 cents a loaf? Or if General Electric adds $100 to the price of a refrigerator? Or if Ford raises the price of a new car by $2,500? Those are all market-based decisions designed to increase a company's financial stability and profitability. So how can drug companies be held to another standard than other corporations? Are they not also entitled to make a fair profit on the goods they product? And, if they *are* so entitled, how can anyone question the legitimacy of rising drug prices?

The response to that question is fairly obvious. Drug companies do not produce items that a consumer would like to have, like a new refrigerator or new car, but substances that they need to stay healthy, treat disease, and even stay alive. Shkreli's company's Daraprim, for example, is one of the few drugs available for the treatment of toxoplasmosis, probably the most widespread parasitic infection in the world. For millions of people, the drug is not a luxury item that they can choose whether to buy: they need it to stay healthy. Somewhat similar arguments can be made with greater or less import about most drugs in pharmacopoeias today.

Given this background, one can see why efforts to deal with drug prices are extraordinarily difficult in the United States, especially in comparison to those in almost all other countries of the world where other economic systems are in effect to one degree or another capitalistic (Hancock 2017). Nonetheless, we continue with a review of some of the most common approaches that have been used to reduce the burdens of ever-increasing prescription drug prices.

One of the most common recommendations for dealing with rising drug prices is to liberalize the U.S. policy of drug *importation* and *reimportation*. These terms refer to the ability of U.S. consumers to purchase their prescription drugs from sources outside the United States. As noted previously, prescription drugs are less expensive in almost every developed country in the world, so it might make some sense if U.S citizens were allowed to buy their drugs from Canada, the United Kingdom, France, Germany, or some other foreign nation. This option has been discussed for at least two decades, with relatively little progress in its implementation. See, for example, Groman (2005).

Today, that policy recommendation has been pared down to include only Canada as a possible source of imported drugs. Studies have shown that drugs imported from Canada cost somewhere between 28 and 35 percent less than identical products in the United States. The conditions under which drug importation from Canada can occur were laid out primarily in two pieces of legislation: the Medicine Equity and Drug Safety Act of 2000 and MMA of 2003. Drugs that can be shipped from Canada to the United States fall into two general categories. The first includes drugs that are (1) manufactured at foreign sites that have been inspected by the FDA, (2) being considered for approval by the FDA, (3) specifically intended for use by U.S. consumers, or (4) imported to the United States by the drug manufacturer. The second category of drugs are those that have been made in the United States, shipped to a foreign country, and then reimported to the United States by the manufacturer (Freed, Neuman, and Cubanski 2020).

A possible step toward implementing drug importation from Canada was announced in December 2019. Under an Executive Order issued by President Donald Trump, the Food and Drug Administration and Department of Health and Human Services (HHS) announced plans to adopt a new rule that would allow states to pass laws allowing drug importations from Canada. At the time the announcement was made, three states had passed laws allowing residents to receive drugs from Canadian suppliers. Two more states passed similar laws after the new rule was announced. Those laws could not go into effect, however, until the federal government adopted regulations allowing them to do so, the reason for the FDA/HHS "new rule" announcement. The whole process will require many steps before becoming a reality and, according to some sources, "it likely will be years before states can actually implement importation plans" (Inserro 2019; Owermohle, Karlin-Smith, and Fineout 2019). Trump's important plans also met with some incredulity from experts in the field, who offered a variety of reasons the plan simply would not work. See, for example, Pipes (2020). One such problem appears to be that Canadian exporters themselves have been rejecting and are likely to reject any opportunity to take part in the plan, that is, to actually ship drugs to the United States (Martell 2019).

Another approach to reducing the rise in drug prices is to adopt legislation allowing the FDA and/or HHS to negotiate with drug manufacturers on drug pricing. Currently, such actions are specifically prohibited by provisions of the Medicare Modernization Act of 2003. The so-called noninterference clause of that Act provides that the HHS secretary "may not interfere with the negotiations between drug manufacturers and pharmacies and PDP sponsors; and (2) may not require a particular formulary or institute a price structure for the reimbursement of covered part D drugs" ("Subpart 2—Prescription Drug Plans; PDP Sponsors; Financing" n.d.). The reason behind this provision is that such actions by a representative of the government would interfere with the normal functioning of the marketplace, preventing competition among companies for the best approach for dealing with drug prices. Traditionally, the Republican party has taken this position on drug negotiation, while Democrats have been more open to allowing government interference.

Over the past two decades, a debate has continued as to whether or not the HHS, FDA, or other federal agency should become involved in the process of drug pricing. The most recent debate has centered on H.R. 3, introduced in the House of Representatives by Frank Pallone (D-NJ) on September 19,

2019. That bill, now known as the Elijah E. Cummings Lower Drug Costs Now Act, passed the House on December 12, 2019, on a largely party-line vote: 230 (all Democrats) to 192 (all but two Republicans). The bill was not considered by the Senate, where it faced substantial opposition by the dominant Republican party.

The votes on H.R. 3 do not represent popular opinion on the importance of drug price negotiations. In one 2017 public opinion poll, 96 percent of all Democrats polled as well as 92 percent of both Republicans and Independents expressed support for some type of governmental action along these lines (Kirzinger, et al. 2017).

H.R. 3 was only one of several cost reduction bills introduced in both the House and the Senate. All bills differ from each other to a greater or lesser degree and, therefore, are likely to have greater or lesser effect on drug prices. The Congressional Budget Office (CBO) estimated that H.R. 3 would have "negligible" effects on drug prices because the secretary of the HHS was still not provided with adequate power to negotiate prices. CBO estimates for other bills, however, are quite different, with savings of up to $345 billion in Medicare drug costs between 2023 and 2029 (Cubanski, et al. 2019).

A somewhat less common suggestion in the United States for dealing with the rising cost of prescription drugs is value-based pricing (VBP), a system described previously. In a VBP plan, the cost of a drug is based not on a pharmaceutical company's own decision as to the monetary value of a drug but on independent determinations of the value it has in treatment of a disease or disorder. The system has been in operation in the European Union for many years, with substantial success. But it has not yet become widely popular in the United States.

One reason for the current lack of interest in VBP is, of course, that drug companies will make less profit on their products than under current systems of pricing. The first challenge in many cases, then, is to get companies to accept reduced profits in exchange for other benefits granted to them by insurance companies, the federal and state governments, and other entities. A second problem with VBP is the nature of the health care system in the United States. So many diverse elements exist (private care providers, insurers, hospitals, state and federal agencies, etc.) that it is difficult to know how to get all entities to agree on the same standards for the "value" of a drug.

Probably the most basic issue is deciding how to determine the monetary value any one drug might have. The problem is less severe, perhaps, for one-disease drugs, such as a drug to treat amyotrophic lateral sclerosis. One might just measure the number of patients whose condition improves by one standard or another and how much financial cost is saved in that way. But the vast majority of drugs cannot be analyzed by that procedure. Any one drug might be used for a variety of disorders by individuals of very different backgrounds under different medical conditions. As a result, everyone involved in establishing a VBP has a host of questions to answer with many stakeholders to set up such a program. There is now a vast literature on VBP and its possible use in the United States. See especially Armstrong and Becker (2019) for state actions on VBPs; "Getting at the Value of Value-Based Drug Pricing Models" (2018), for an overview of some methods that have been used to measure drug value; "Value-Based Pricing for Prescription Drugs: Opportunities and Challenges" (2016), for a transcript of a podcast with stakeholders having a special interest and expertise in VBP; Coughlin (2019), for a description of a new Massachusetts program for assessing drug values; Goldman and Jena (2017), for a review of specific problems relating to the development of VBP programs; and Chapman, et al. (2019), for a most thorough and extensive discussion of all aspects of the use of VBP in the United States.

Additional suggestions include the following: ("American Patients First" 2018 [then president Trump's list of twenty-eight ways of reducing prescription drug costs], Augustine, Madhavan, and Nass 2018, Twomey 2019):

- speeding approval of cheaper generics
- requiring notification by drug companies before they raise prices
- restricting drug ads aimed at consumers
- banning patents for pills that simply modify existing medicines without significant clinical benefits

Conclusion

The invention, development, and use of prescription drugs have been one of the most important breakthroughs in the history of medicine. These substances have relieved pain, cured disease, aided in the cure of other disorders and, generally, extended and saved the lives of a countless number of humans around the world over the past century. But the availability of prescription drugs has come not without its own set of challenges and problems. For example, the development and use of prescription drugs has traditionally followed a one-size-fits-all model, an assumption that any one drug will have all—or nearly all—the same effects on all individuals, no matter their sex, race, ethnic background, or other personal characteristic. Today, drug researchers are taking a more informed view of this philosophy and developing more diversified tests for new drugs.

The availability of prescription drugs has also vastly increased the possibility of drug abuse and a host of medical, social, economic, and other problems associated with this issue. Finally, perhaps the most discussed issue today is the seemingly ever-increasing costs of prescription drugs, a problem of substantially serious concern to Americans of virtually every economic level. Politicians, government officials, researchers, and other stakeholders are now focusing more on how this problem has developed and how it can be solved in coming years.

References

"ACLU Asks Court to Protect Confidentiality of Rush Limbaugh's Medical Records." 2004. American Civil Liberties Union. https://www.aclu.org/news/aclu-asks-court-protect-confidentiality-rush-limbaughs-medical-records.

Alogailia, Fahdm, Norjihan Abdul Ghania, and Nordiana Ahmad Kharman Shahb. 2020. "Prescription Drug Monitoring Programs in the US: A Systematic Literature Review on Its Strength and Weakness." *Journal of Infection and Public Health*. https://doi.org/10.1016/j.jiph.2020.06.035.

Alter, Aliese, and Christopher Yeager. 2020. "COVID-19 Impact on US National Overdose Crisis." Overdose Detection Mapping Application Program. http://www.odmap.org/Content/docs/news/2020/ODMAP-Report-June-2020.pdf.

"American Patients First." 2018. Secretary of Health and Human Services. https://www.hhs.gov/sites/default/files/AmericanPatientsFirst.pdf.

Anderson, Richard. 2014. "Pharmaceutical Industry Gets High on Fat Profits." BBC News. https://www.bbc.com/news/business-28212223.

"Animal Welfare Act." n.d. National Agricultural Library, U.S. Department of Agriculture. https://www.nal.usda.gov/awic/animal-welfare-act.

"The Animal Welfare Act." Public Law 89-544. 1966. https://www.govinfo.gov/content/pkg/STATUE-80-Pg350.pdf.

"Animal Welfare Act Timeline." n.d. Animal Welfare Act History Digital Collection, U.S. Department of Agriculture. https://awahistory.nal.usda.gov/timeline/list.

Armstrong, John, and Colleen Becker. 2019. "Value-Based Pricing to Address Drug Costs." Our American States.

National Conference of State Legislatures. 27(15). https://www.ncsl.org/research/health/value-based-pricing-to-address-drug-costs.aspx.

Arnold, John. 2018. "Are Pharmacy Benefit Managers the Good Guys or Bad Guys of Drug Pricing?" Stat. https://www.statnews.com/2018/08/27/pharmacy-benefit-managers-good-or-bad/.

Augustine, Norman R., Guruprasad Madhavan, and Sharyl J. Nass, eds. 2018. *Making Medicines Affordable: A National Imperative.* Washington, D.C.: National Academies Press.

Bao, Yuhua, et al. 2016. "Prescription Drug Monitoring Programs Are Associated with Sustained Reductions in Opioid Prescribing By Physicians." *Health Affairs.* 35(6): 1045–1051. https://doi.org/10.1377/hlthaff.2015.1673.

Barrell, Amanda. 2019. "How to Address Racial Disparities in Clinical Trial Data." pharmaphorum. https://pharmaphorum.com/views-analysis-patients/utilising-technology-racial-disparities-clinical-trial-data/.

Bever, Lindsey. 2018. "A Town of 3,200 Was Flooded with Nearly 21 Million Pain Pills as Addiction Crisis Worsened, Lawmakers Say." *The Washington Post.* https://www.washingtonpost.com/news/to-your-health/wp/2018/01/31/a-town-of-3200-was-flooded-with-21-million-pain-pills-as-addiction-crisis-worsened-lawmakers-say/.

Bonaime, Alice A., and Ye (Emma) Wang. 2020. "Mergers, Product Prices, and Innovation: Evidence from the Pharmaceutical Industry." SSRN. http://dx.doi.org/10.2139/ssrn.3445753.

Brande, Lauren. 2020. "Effects of Stimulant Drugs." Drugabuse.com. https://drugabuse.com/stimulants/effects-use/.

Brennan, Zachary. 2019. "Do Biopharma Companies Really Spend More on Marketing than R&D?" Regulatory Focus. https://www.raps.org/news-and-articles/news-articles/2019/7/do-biopharma-companies-really-spend-more-on-market.

Castle, Grant, Brian Kelly, and Raj Gathani. 2020. "Pricing & Reimbursement 2020 United Kingdom." Global Legal Insights. https://www.globallegalinsights.com/practice-areas/pricing-and-reimbursement-laws-and-regulations/united-kingdom.

Chapman, Rick, et al. 2019. "Value Assessment Methods and Pricing Recommendations for Potential Cures: A Technical Brief." Institute for Clinical and Economic Review. https://icer-review.org/wp-content/uploads/2019/08/ICER_TechnicalBrief_SSTs_080619-1.pdf.

Chen, Caroline, and Riley Wong. 2018. "Black Patients Miss Out on Promising Cancer Drugs." ProPublica. https://www.propublica.org/article/black-patients-miss-out-on-promising-cancer-drugs.

Claxton, Karl, Mark J. Sculpher, and Stuart Carroll. 2011. "Value-Based Pricing for Pharmaceuticals: Its Role, Specification, and Prospects in a Newly Devolved NHS." York, UK: Centre for Health Economics. University of York. https://www.york.ac.uk/media/che/documents/papers/researchpapers/CHERP60_value_based_pricing_for_pharmaceuticals.pdf.

Clifford, Stephanie. 2018. "Martin Shkreli Sentenced to 7 Years in Prison for Fraud." *The New York Times*. https://www.nytimes.com/2018/03/09/business/martin-shkreli-sentenced.html.

"Combat Addiction and Become the Man You Were Meant to Be." 2015. Recovery Boot Camp. https://www.recoverybootcamp.com/oxycontin-addiction-treatment/.

Conner, Annastasia. 2017. "Galen's Analogy: Animal Experimentation and Anatomy in the Second Century C.E." *Anthós*. 8(1): Article 9. doi: 10.15760/anthos.2017.118.

Coughlin, Bob. 2019. "How Do You Measure the Real Value of Prescription Drugs?" MassBio. https://www.massbio

.org/news/recent-news/how-do-you-measure-the-real-value-of-prescription-drugs/.

Cubanski, Juliette, et al. 2019. "What's the Latest on Medicare Drug Price Negotiations?" Kaiser Family Foundation. https://www.kff.org/medicare/issue-brief/whats-the-latest-on-medicare-drug-price-negotiations/.

"Data Brief 394. 2020. Drug Overdose Deaths in the United States, 1999–2019." https://www.cdc.gov/nchs/data/databriefs/db394-tables-508.pdf#page=1.

"Doctor Shopping Laws." 2012. Centers for Disease Control and Prevention. http://www.cdc.gov/phlp/docs/menu-shoppinglaws.pdf.

Drug Enforcement Administration. 2020. "Quick Links." https://search.dea.gov/search.

"Drug Pricing." 2010. PostNote. Houses of Parliament. https://www.parliament.uk/documents/post/postpn_364_Drug_Pricing.pdf.

Dunn, Andrew, and Ned Pagliarulo. 2019. "Follow the Money: How Biopharma CEOs and Workers Got Paid in 2018." Biopharmadive. https://www.biopharmadive.com/news/biotech-pharma-ceo-employee-pay/554283/.

Elhadi, Ali M., et al. 2012. "The Journey of Discovering Skull Base Anatomy in Ancient Egypt and the Special Influence of Alexandria." *Neurosurgical Focus*. 33(2): E2. doi: 10.3171/2012.6.FOCUS12128

"Fatal Drug Overdoses Hit a Record High Last Year. Covid-19 Is Making the Problem Worse." 2020. Advisory Board. https://www.advisory.com/daily-briefing/2020/07/17/overdose.

"Fentanyl Drug Facts." 2019. National Institute on Drug Abuse. https://www.drugabuse.gov/publications/drugfacts/fentanyl.

"Florida's Prescription Drug Diversion and Abuse Roadmap 2012–2015." 2012. http://www.flsenate.gov/Session/Bill/2011/7095/BillText/er/PDF.

"45-9-104. Fraudulently Obtaining Dangerous Drugs."
2017. Montana Code Annotated 2017. http://leg.mt
.gov/bills/mca/title_0450/chapter_0090/part_0010/
section_0040/0450-0090-0010-0040.html.

Fralick, Michael, and Aaron S. Kesselheim. 2019. "The
U.S. Insulin Crisis—Rationing a Lifesaving Medication
Discovered in the 1920s." *New England Journal of
Medicine.* 381:1793–1795. doi: 10.1056/NEJMp1909402.

Franco, Nuno Henrique. 2013. "Animal Experiments in
Biomedical Research: A Historical Perspective." *Animals.*
3(1): 238–273. doi: 10.3390/ani3010238.

Franconi, Flavia, et al. 2019. "Sex–Gender Variable:
Methodological Recommendations for Increasing Scientific
Value of Clinical Studies." *Cells.* 8(5): 476. doi: 10.3390/
cells8050476.

Freed, Meredith, Tricia Neuman, and Juliette Cubanski.
2020. "10 FAQs on Prescription Drug Importation."
Kaiser Family Foundation. https://www.kff.org/medicare/
issue-brief/10-faqs-on-prescription-drug-importation/

Garrett, Jeremy R. 2012. *The Ethics of Animal Research:
Exploring the Controversy.* Cambridge, MA: MIT Press.

"Getting at the Value of Value–Based Drug Pricing
Models." 2018. Pharmaceutical Commerce. https://
pharmaceuticalcommerce.com/brand-marketing-
communications/getting-at-the-value-of-value-
based-drug-pricing-models/.

Goldman, Dana, and Anupam B. Jena. 2017. "Value–
Based Drug Pricing Makes Sense, but Is Difficult to
Pull off." Stat. https://www.statnews.com/2017/06/08/
value-based-drug-pricing/.

Goliszek, Andrew. 2011. *In the Name of Science: A History
of Secret Programs, Medical Research, and Human
Experimentation.* New York: St. Martin's Press.

Groman, Rachel. 2005. "Prescription Drug Importation as
a Policy Option to Lower the Cost of Medications in the

U.S." American College of Physicians. https://www
.acponline.org/acp_policy/policies/presdrug_import_
policy_option_lower_cost_medications_2006.pdf.

Guerrini, Anita. 2003. *Experimenting with Humans and
Animals: From Galen to Animal Rights.* Baltimore, MD: The
Johns Hopkins University Press.

"Guideline for the Format and Content of the Nonclinical
Pharmacology/Toxicology Section of an Application."
1987. U.S. Food and Drug Administration. https://www
.fda.gov/media/72223/download.

Hancock, Jay. 2017. "Everyone Wants to Reduce Drug
Prices. So Why Can't We Do It?" *The New York Times.*
https://www.nytimes.com/2017/09/23/sunday-review/
prescription-drugs-prices.html.

"Harold Rogers Prescription Drug Monitoring Program."
2010. Bureau of Justice Assistance. https://www
.deadiversion.usdoj.gov/mtgs/drug_chemical/2010/
rrose.pdf.

Herman, Bob. 2018. "Pharma's Grip on the Health Care
Economy." Axios. https://www.axios.com/pharma-health-
care-economy-q3-profits-53b950b2-5515-4d79-b1f5-
7067bf3652d1.html.

Hernandez, Immaculada, et al. 2019. "The Contribution of
New Product Entry Versus Existing Product Inflation in
the Rising Costs of Drugs." *Health Affairs.* 38(1). https://
doi.org/10.1377/hlthaff.2018.05147.

Herrera, Angelica P., et al. 2010. "Disparate Inclusion
of Older Adults in Clinical Trials: Priorities and
Opportunities for Policy and Practice Change." *American
Journal of Public Health.* 100(Suppl 1): S105–S112. doi:
10.2105/AJPH.2009.162982.

"Highlights of Prescribing Information." 2017. U.S. Food
and Drug Administration. https://www.accessdata.fda.gov/
drugsatfda_docs/label/2017/209777lbl.pdf.

Hoff, Caitlin. 2019. "Taking on Gender Bias in Clinical Trials." National Women's Health Network. https://nwhn.org/taking-on-gender-bias-in-clinical-trials/.

Inserro, Allison. 2019. "US Unveils Proposed Rules to Allow Some Canadian Drug Imports." AJMC. https://www.ajmc.com/view/us-unveils-proposed-rules-to-allow-some-canadian-drug-imports.

"Institutional Review Boards: Frequently Asked Questions." 1998/2019. U.S. Food and Drug Administration. https://www.fda.gov/regulatory-information/search-fda-guidance-documents/institutional-review-boards-frequently-asked-questions.

Keefe, Patrick Radden. 2017. "The Family That Built an Empire of Pain." *The New Yorker*. https://www.newyorker.com/magazine/2017/10/30/the-family-that-built-an-empire-of-pain.

Keenan, Colleen. 2020. "How Covid-19 Is Impacting the Opioid Crisis (And 5 Ways Providers Can Help)." Advisory Board. https://www.advisory.com/daily-briefing/2020/06/10/opioids-covid.

Kennedy-Hendricks, Alene, et al. 2016. "Opioid Overdose Deaths and Florida's Crackdown on Pill Mills." *American Journal of Public Health*. 106(2): 291–297. doi: 10.2105/AJPH.2015.302953.

Khan, Muchammad Shahzeb, et al. 2020. "Ten Year Trends in Enrollment of Women and Minorities in Pivotal Trials Supporting Recent US Food and Drug Administration Approval of Novel Cardiometabolic Drugs." *Journal of the American Heart Association*. 9(11): 9. https://doi.org/10.1161/JAHA.119.015594.

Kirzinger, Ashley, et al. 2017. "Kaiser Health Tracking Poll—Late April 2017: The Future of the ACA and Health Care & the Budget." Kaiser Family Foundation. https://www.kff.org/report-section/.

kaiser-health-tracking-poll-late-april-2017-the-future-of-the-aca-and-health-care-the-budget-rx-drugs/.

Kirzinger, Ashley, et al. 2019. "KFF Health Tracking Poll—February 2019: Prescription Drugs." Kaiser Family Foundation. https://www.kff.org/health-costs/poll-finding/kff-health-tracking-poll-february-2019-prescription-drugs/.

Kodjak, Alison 2019. "Prescription Drug Costs Driven by Manufacturer Price Hikes, Not Innovation." NPR. https://www.npr.org/sections/health-shots/2019/01/07/682986630/prescription-drug-costs-driven-by-manufacturer-price-hikes-not-innovation.

Kunzmann, Kevin, and Kenny Walter. 2020. "The 3 Waves of the Opioid Epidemic." HCP Live. https://www.hcplive.com/view/3-waves-opioid-epidemic.

Lakhan, Shaheen E., and Annette Kirchgessner. 2012. "Prescription Stimulants in Individuals with and without Attention Deficit Hyperactivity Disorder: Misuse, Cognitive Impact, and Adverse Effects." *Brain and Behavior.* 2(5): 661–677. http://www.ncbi.nlm.nih.gov/pmc/articles/PMC3489818/.

Lennox, James. 2011. "Aristotle's Biology." *The Stanford Encyclopedia of Philosophy* (Fall 2011 edition). http://plato.stanford.edu/archives/fall2011/entries/aristotle-biology/.

Liu, Katherine A., and Natalie A. Dipietro Mager. 2016. "Women's Involvement in Clinical Trials: Historical Perspective and Future Implications." *Pharmacology Practice.* 14(1): 708. doi: 10.18549/PharmPract.2016.01.708.

"A Look at Drug Spending in the U.S." 2018. Pew. https://www.pewtrusts.org/en/research-and-analysis/fact-sheets/2018/02/a-look-at-drug-spending-in-the-us.

Luo, Jing, Jerry Avorn, and Aaron S. Kesselheim. 2015. "Trends in Medicaid Reimbursements for Insulin from 1991 through 2014." *JAMA Internal*

Medicine. 175(10):1681–1686. doi: 10.1001/
jamainternmed.2015.4338.

Luxner, Larry. 2019. "Debate Shifts to Pricing and Availability
of World's Costliest Drug." *SMA News Today.* https://
smanewstoday.com/2019/05/29/zolgensma-approval-shifts-
debate-pricing-availability-worlds-costliest-drug/.

"Making Use of Your State's Prescription Drug Monitoring
Program." 2020. Search and Rescue. https://
searchandrescueusa.org/monitoryourpatients/.

"Market Share of the Top 5 Pharmacy Benefit Managers in
the U.S. Prescription Market in 2018." 2020. Statista.
https://www.statista.com/statistics/239976/us-prescription-
market-share-of-top-pharmacy-benefit-managers/.

Marsh, Tori. 2018. "2 Years after the EpiPen Price Hike,
Here's What's Changed." GoodRx. https://www.goodrx
.com/blog/epipen-price-change-since-mylan-released-
generic-epinephrine/.

Marsh, Tori. 2020a. "Live Updates: January Drug Price
Hikes Are Here." GoodRx. https://www.goodrx.com/blog/
january-drug-price-hikes-2020/.

Marsh, Tori. 2020b. "Live Updates: July 2020 Drug Price
Increases." GoodRx. https://www.goodrx.com/blog/
july-drug-price-hikes-2020/.

Martell, Allison. 2019. "Canadian Drug Distributors
Say No to Trump Import Plan." Reuters. https://www
.reuters.com/article/us-usa-healthcare-canada/canadian-
drug-distributors-say-no-to-trump-import-plan-
idUSKBN1YO24O.

Mayo Clinic. 2019. "Understanding the Risks of Performance-
Enhancing Drugs." www.mayoclinic.org/healthy-life
style/fitness/in-depth/performance-enhancing-drugs/
art-20046134.

McCarthy, C. R. 1994. "Historical Background of Clinical
Trials Involving Women and Minorities." *Academic*

Medicine. 69(9): 695–698. doi: 10.1097/00001888-199409000-00002.

"Measuring Prescription Drug Prices: A Primer on the CPI Prescription Drug Index." 2019. https://www.ssr health.com/wp-content/uploads/2019/10/2019_CEA_Measuring-Prescription-Drug-Prices-A-Primer-on-the-CPI-Prescription-Drug-Index.pdf.

"Medicines in Development for Cell Therapy and Gene Therapy." 2018. Medicines in Development 2018 Report. http://phrma-docs.phrma.org/files/dmfile/MID_Cell_and_Gene_Therapy_2018_FINAL.pdf.

Meier, Barry. 2003. *Pain Killer: A "Wonder" Drug's Trail of Addiction and Death.* Emmaus, PA: Rodale.

Meier, Barry. 2018. *Pain Killer: An Empire of Deceit and the Origin of America's Opioid Epidemic.* New York: Random House.

Merkatz, R. B. 1998. "Inclusion of Women in Clinical Trials: A Historical Overview of Scientific, Ethical, and Legal Issues." *Journal of Obstetrics, Gynecology, and Neonatal Nursing.* 27(1): 78–84. doi: 10.1111/j.1552-6909.1998.tb02594.x.

"Mice and Rats in Laboratories." 2020. People for the Ethical Treatment of Animals. https://www.peta.org/issues/animals-used-for-experimentation/animals-laboratories/mice-rats-laboratories.

Miller, Michael E. 2015. "Pharma Bro' Martin Shkreli and the Very American Debate over Maximizing Profit." *The Washington Post.* https://www.washingtonpost.com/news/morning-mix/wp/2015/09/23/pharma-bro-martin-shkreli-and-the-very-american-debate-over-maximizing-profit/.

"Misuse of Prescription Drugs Research Report." 2020. National Institute on Drug Abuse. https://www.drugabuse.gov/download/37630/misuse-prescription-drugs-research-report.pdf.

National Academies of Sciences, Engineering, and Medicine, et al. 2017. "Trends in Opioid Use, Harms, and Treatment." In J. K. Phillips, M. A. Ford, and R. J. Bonnie, eds. *Pain Management and the Opioid Epidemic: Balancing Societal and Individual Benefits and Risks of Prescription Opioid Use*. Washington, D.C.: National Academies Press. https://www.ncbi.nlm.nih.gov/books/NBK458661/.

"National Health Expenditures 2018 Highlights." 2020. Centers for Medicare and Medicaid Services. https://www.cms.gov/files/document/highlights.pdf.

Nazha, Bassel, et al. 2019. "Enrollment of Racial Minorities in Clinical Trials: Old Problem Assumes New Urgency in the Age of Immunotherapy." *American Society of Clinical Oncology Educational Book*. 39: 3–10. doi: 10.1200/EDBK_100021.

"New Drug Pricing Analysis Reveals Where PBMs and Pharmacies Make Their Money." 2019. 46brooklyn. https://www.46brooklyn.com/research/2019/4/21/new-pricing-data-reveals-where-pbms-and-pharmacies-make-their-money.

Newport, Frank. 2020. "Public Opinion Review: Americans' Reactions to the Word 'Socialism.'" Gallup. https://news.gallup.com/opinion/polling-matters/287459/public-opinion-review-americans-word-socialism.aspx.

Newton, David E. 2013. *The Animal Experimentation Debate: A Reference Handbook*. Santa Barbara, CA: ABC-CLIO.

Newton, David E. 2018. *The Opioid Crisis*. Santa Barbara, CA: ABC-CLIO.

"The Next U.S. Drug Epidemic As of 2019." 2020. Keck School of Medicine of USC. https://mphdegree.usc.edu/blog/the-next-u-s-drug-epidemic-as-of-2019/.

"NIH Policy and Guidelines on the Inclusion of Women and Minorities as Subjects in Clinical Research." 2017. NIH Grants & Funding. https://grants.nih.gov/policy/inclusion/women-and-minorities/guidelines.htm.

Nowogrodzki, Anna. 2017. "Inequality in Medicine." *Nature.* 550(7674): S18–S19. https://doi.org/10.1038/550S18a.

Ohler, Norman. 2015. *Blitzed: Drugs in the Third Reich.* Boston: Houghton Mifflin Harcourt.

The Opioid Epidemic: Tracking a Crisis. 2019. New York Times Educational Publishing.

O'Reilly, Eileen Drage, and Alison Snyder. 2020. "The Cost of Racial Disparities in Clinical Trials." Axios. https://www.axios.com/black-americans-diseases-clinical-trials-2acaa476-0ec8-4362-8e90-2f5c3c85c916.html.

"Overpatented, Overpriced: How Excessive Pharmaceutical Patenting Is Extending Monopolies and Driving Up Drug Prices." 2018. I·MAK. http://www.i-mak.org/wp-content/uploads/2018/08/I-MAK-Overpatented-Overpriced-Report.pdf.

Owermohle, Sarah, Sarah Karlin-Smith, and Gary Fineout. 2019. "Trump Plan Would Allow States to Import Drugs from Canada." Politico. https://www.politico.com/news/2019/12/18/trump-states-import-canadian-drugs-086918.

"PBM Companies." 2020. shortlister. https://www.myshortlister.com/pbm-companies/vendor-list.

Perry, Samuel, and George Heidrich. 1982. "Management of Pain during Debridement: A Survey of U.S. Burn Units." *Pain.* 13(3): 267–280.

"Pharmaceutical Spending per Capita in Selected Countries as of 2018." 2020. Statista. https://www.statista.com/statistics/266141/pharmaceutical-spending-per-capita-in-selected-countries/.

"Pill Mill Initiative." 2011. Florida Office of the Attorney General. http://myfloridalegal.com/pages.nsf/Main/AA7AAF5CAA22638D8525791B006A30C8.

Piper, Brian J., et al. 2016. "Trends in Use of Prescription Stimulants in the United States and Territories, 2006 to 2016." *PloS One.* 13(11): e0206100. doi:10.1371/journal.pone.0206100.

Pipes, Sally. "The Epic Folly of Trump's Drug Importation Crusade." 2020. Forbes. https://www.forbes.com/sites/ sallypipes/2020/01/06/the-epic-folly-of-trumps-drug-importation-crusade/#550eb5a9753d.

"Policy Changes Could Bolster Prescription Drug Monitoring Programs." 2020. Pew. https://www.pewtrusts.org/en/ research-and-analysis/issue-briefs/2020/04/policy-changes-could-bolster-prescription-drug-monitoring-programs.

Porter, Jane, and Hershel Jick. 1980. "Addiction Rare in Patients Treated with Narcotics." *New England Journal of Medicine.* 302(2): 123. http://www.nejm.org/doi/ pdf/10.1056/NEJM198001103020221.

Prasad, Vinay, and Sham Mailankody. 2017. "Research and Development Spending to Bring a Single Cancer Drug to Market and Revenues after Approval." *JAMA Internal Medicine.* 177(11): 1569–1575.

"Prescription Drug Expenditures; Aggregate and Per Capita Amounts, Percent Distribution and Annual Percent Change by Source of Funds; Calendar Years 2011–2027." 2020. Centers for Medicare and Medicaid. https://www .cms.gov/Research-Statistics-Data-and-Systems/Statistics-Trends-and-Reports/NationalHealthExpendData/ NationalHealthAccountsProjected.

"Prescription Drug Spending in the U.S. Health Care System." 2018. American Academy of Actuaries. https://www.actuary.org/content/prescription-drug-spending-us-health-care-system.

"Prescription Sedatives (Tranquilizers, Sedatives)." 2016. Facing Addiction in America: The Surgeon General's Report on Alcohol, Drugs, and Health. https://www.ncbi .nlm.nih.gov/books/NBK424847/table/appd.t15/.

"Regulations, Guidance, and Reports Related to Women's Health." 2019. U.S. Food and Drug Administration. https://www.fda.gov/science-research/womens-health-research/ regulations-guidance-and-reports-related-womens-health.

"Research Facility Annual Summary & Archive Reports." 2020. Animal and Plant Health Inspection Service, U.S. Department of Agriculture. https://www.aphis.usda.gov/aphis/ourfocus/animalwelfare/sa_obtain_research_facility_annual_report/ct_research_facility_annual_summary_reports.

Reverby, Susan M. 2009. *Examining Tuskegee: The Infamous Syphilis Study and Its Legacy*. Chapel Hill, NC: University of North Carolina Press.

Rochon, Paul A., Philip B. Berger, and Michael Gordon. 1998. "The Evolution of Clinical Trials: Inclusion and Representation." CMAJ. 159(11): 1373–1374. https://www.cmaj.ca/content/cmaj/159/11/1373.full.pdf.

Sanneh, Kelefa. 2016. "Everyone Hates Martin Shkreli. Everyone Is Missing the Point." *The New Yorker*. https://www.newyorker.com/culture/cultural-comment/everyone-hates-martin-shkreli-everyone-is-missing-the-point.

Sarnak, Dana O., David Squires, and Shawn Bishop. 2017. "Paying for Prescription Drugs around the World: Why Is the U.S. an Outlier?" The Commonwealth Fund. https://www.commonwealthfund.org/publications/issue-briefs/2017/oct/paying-prescription-drugs-around-world-why-us-outlier.

Schneberg, Todd, et al. 2020. "Opioid Prescription Patterns among Patients Who Doctor Shop; Implications for Providers." *PLoS One*. 15(5): e0232533. doi: 10.1371/journal.pone.0232533.

Schwartzapfel, Beth. 2017. "Guess Who's Tracking Your Prescription Drugs." *The Marshall Project*. https://www.themarshallproject.org/2017/08/02/guess-whos-tracking-your-prescription-drugs.

Scott, Jim. 2019. "Chairman's Blog: Underrepresentation of Older Adults in Clinical Trials." Alliance for Aging

Research. https://www.agingresearch.org/chairmans-blog-underrepresentation-of-older-adults-in-clinical-trials/.

Shah, Parth, et al. 2020. "Informed Consent." StatPearls. https://www.ncbi.nlm.nih.gov/books/NBK430827/.

Sharav, Vera Hassner. 2010. "Human Experiments: A Chronology of Human Research." Alliance for Human Research Protection. https://web.archive.org/web/20100502075736/http://www.ahrp.org/history/chronology.php.

Shea, Jonathan N. 2019. "Is There Really a Difference between Drug Addiction and Drug Dependence?" *Scientific American.* https://blogs.scientificamerican.com/observations/is-there-really-a-difference-between-drug-addiction-and-drug-dependence/.

"Should Animals Be Used for Scientific or Commercial Testing?" 2020. Britannia ProCon.org. https://animal-testing.procon.org/.

"Significant Changes in Drug Use during the Pandemic." 2020. Millennium Health Signals Report. https://resource.millenniumhealth.com/signalsreportCOVID.

"Study and Evaluation of Gender Differences in the Clinical Evaluation of Drugs." 2020. U.S. Food and Drug Administration. https://www.fda.gov/regulatory-information/search-fda-guidance-documents/study-and-evaluation-gender-differences-clinical-evaluation-drugs.

"Subpart 2—Prescription Drug Plans; PDP Sponsors; Financing." n.d. Social Security. https://www.ssa.gov/OP_Home/ssact/title18/1860D-11.htm.

Taylor, Phil. 2020. "The Top 10 Pharma R&D Budgets in 2019." Fierce Biotech. https://www.fiercebiotech.com/special-report/top-10-pharma-r-d-budgets-2019.

Taylor, Timothy. 2019. "Prescription Drug Prices Are Falling (Says the Consumer Price Index)." Conversable Economist.

https://conversableeconomist.blogspot.com/2019/12/
prescription-drug-prices-are-falling.html.

"TED: The Economics Daily." 2020. U.S. Bureau of Labor
Statistics. https://www.bls.gov/opub/ted/2020/consumer-
prices-increase-2-point-5-percent-in-the-12-months-
ending-january-2020.htm.

Teter, Christian J., and Sally K. Guthrie. 2001.
"A Comprehensive Review of MDMA and GHB: Two
Common Club Drugs." *Pharmacotherapy* 21 (12): 1486–
1513. https://doi.org/10.1592/phco.21.20.1486.34472.

"Thalidomide." 2019. Science Museum. https://www
.sciencemuseum.org.uk/objects-and-stories/medicine/
thalidomide.

Tikkanen, Roosa, and Melinda K. Abrams. 2020. "U.S.
Health Care from a Global Perspective, 2019: Higher
Spending, Worse Outcomes?" The Commonwealth
Fund. https://www.commonwealthfund.org/publications/
issue-briefs/2020/jan/us-health-care-global-
perspective-2019.

"Title 16, Health and Safety, Food and Drugs." 2017.
Controlled Substances Act, Chapter 47, Subchapter IV.
Offenses and Penalties. State of Delaware. http://www
.delcode.delaware.gov/title16/c047/sc04/index.shtml.

"Transforming Lives, Advancing Hope." 2019. 2019
Janssen U.S. Transparency Report. https://jnj-janssen
.brightspotcdn.com/19/3f/55f6149249348ab7c64ba8
81c638/jsn-2019-us-transparency-report-v16.pdf.

"2019 Drug Trials Snapshots. Summary Report." 2020. U.S.
Food and Drug Administration. https://www.fda.gov/
media/135337/download.

Twomey, Madeline. 2019. "Comprehensive Reform to Lower
Prescription Drug Prices." Center for American Progress.
https://www.americanprogress.org/issues/healthcare/
news/2019/01/29/465621/comprehensive-reform-lower-
prescription-drug-prices/.

Unger, Joseph M., et al. 2013. "Patient Income Level and Cancer Clinical Trial Participation." *Journal of Clinical Oncology*. 31(5): 536–542. doi: 10.1200/ JCO.2012.45.4553.

Unger, Joseph M., et al. 2016. "The Role of Clinical Trial Participation in Cancer Research: Barriers, Evidence, and Strategies." *American Society of Clinical Oncology Educational Book*. 36: 185–198. doi: 10.14694/ EDBK_156686.

U.S. Food and Drug Administration. 1993. "FDA Guidance Study and Evaluation of Gender Differences in the Clinical Evaluation of Drugs." Rockville, MD: U.S. Food and Drug Administration.

"U.S. Opioid Prescribing Rate Maps." 2020. Centers for Disease Control and Prevention. https://www.cdc.gov/ drugoverdose/maps/rxrate-maps.html.

"Value-Based Pricing for Prescription Drugs: Opportunities and Challenges." 2016. Alliance for Health Reform. https://www.allhealthpolicy.org/wp-content/ uploads/2016/12/FINALTRANSCRIPT_HM.pdf.

Van Zee, Art. 2009. "The Promotion and Marketing of OxyContin: Commercial Triumph, Public Health Tragedy." *American Journal of Public Health*. 99(2): 221–227. https:// www.ncbi.nlm.nih.gov/pmc/articles/PMC2622774/.

Willingham, Emily. 2016. "Why Did Mylan Hike EpiPen Prices 400%? Because They Could." Forbes. https://www. forbes.com/sites/emilywillingham/2016/08/21/why-did- mylan-hike-epipen-prices-400-because-they-could/.

C 65162-**416**-03

uprenorphine
nd Naloxone
ublingual Tablets

mg*/0.5 mg*

ARMACIST: PLEASE DISPENSE
H MEDICATION GUIDE
OVIDED SEPARATELY

Rx only

30 TABLETS

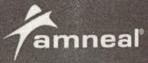

Introduction

The topic of prescription drug inspires responses, ideas, thoughts, and feelings among many individuals. This chapter provides a selection of essays dealing with the topic. The essays range from relatively academic and technical reviews of important issues in the field to personal accounts of one's specific experience in dealing with prescription drugs.

The Cork Board

Kyle Citrin, Clay Knibbs, and Carter Soboleski

Money, relationships, family, loved ones, work, motives, habits, and much more are all daily needs in today's world. A merely invisible force—the force of addiction—acts on much more people than presumed. Each of these living needs becomes corrupt in some fashion by opioid addiction. Priorities become reversed, motives become diminished, and mind-sets become dependent. Someone around you at any moment could be fighting the vigorous attraction of addiction. This attraction is very silent and sometimes undetectable at first, especially from someone close to you. A simple ask of "are you okay?" could be the most piercing sound to one who is under the spell of constant addiction. Once, as he grew up, I saw my older

Naloxone is widely used for the treatment of opioid addiction. (Simone Hogan/Dreamstime.com)

cousin transform from being my fun-loving friend to a rather scary stranger. This path to darkness controls everyone who "chooses" to enter. I saw it in my cousin at a young age but was not completely sure what was happening. I would hear stories of him punching holes through walls when he was upset or treating his mother with utter disrespect. I saw this in my cousin who lived in Atlanta, Georgia, where I only saw him once every couple of years, yet it still took a toll on me and the rest of the family.

The pain occurring inside of a victim's head is often kept quiet, which is kept that way, until it is too late. Not only is an addict constantly in need of a fix, it distracts one from what is truly important in one's life. A situation where one would usually be around his or her sibling/loved one without thought is the same situation where an addiction makes that decision exponentially harder. Thinking twice about drugs becomes turned around into the path of a cruel and never-ending world. The outsider perspective of opioids, and drug addiction in general, is always to stay away from it as much as possible. But once those premises are entered, the lens seemingly gets switched immediately to one that denies exit to anyone who has entered. The entering looks like it would be insanely relieving, but that in itself is the mind trap that gets teenagers in today's world.

What is crazy about it all is that people know this is a concurring event, but no one likes to talk about it. Even when the media gives attention to the staggering statistics around the epidemic, the attention is minimal.

The YouTube video that we made, titled *The Cork Board,* provides not only a visualization of the horrible consequences of an opioid addiction but also the ripple effect that it can have on the victim's loved ones. This is often a troublesome topic to understand for someone who has never experienced the long battle that an addiction can have on someone. Although brief, sixty seconds is all that was required in the video to exhibit the ripple effects of opioids. Shattered relationships, financial hardship, and constant unhappiness are a surface-level viewpoint of the true effects. Seemingly for a user, there is no exit, and no simple way around the addiction. Addiction dictates the actions, emotions, and your entire thought process just from the detrimental action of ingesting a pill.

A user's greatest weapon against addiction and eventual death is the people who surround them. Surrounding yourself with people of similar thinking is often sought after by many, as they can provide support and information that one seeks. Having a clear-minded support system is crucial in the process of becoming clean. An addict is no longer the same person, and with the mind being controlled, addicts see family as none other than someone to exploit in an effort to get more drugs. Addicts will fight and hate you for not providing them money or destroying any drugs they have, as their vision of the greater good has been completely lost.

It is entirely necessary for our society today to educate the youth on these horrifying truths that people struggle with. This means going deeper than having a discussion about drug prevention in a school health class. At this point, it should be less of an informational session and more of an actual demonstration of the horrifying effects pills have. Drug use is normalized in a way in today's society, with rappers in the industry glorifying the highs they get, which in turn leads to the youth listening to the music and thinking drug use is cool. It needs to be seen as less of a trend and more of a life-threatening monster.

Illustrating facts and statistics is crucial to describing the greater issue of prescription drug abuse. Data show the true scale of the problem and allow society to gage the progress regarding the issue. However, a statistical approach is not the solution toward relieving a victim of a prescription drug addiction. When constructing the opioid addiction public service announcement titled *The Cork Board*, the goal was to get personal.

Relationships are considered the most important aspect in life and have a tremendous effect on crucial decisions an individual will make throughout his or her lifetime. In regard to the exploitations of prescription drugs, the harsh reality is that addiction affects more than just the abuser. The worst part is that the addicted user may never realize it until it is too late. When individuals begin the initial steps of drug abuse, they feel as though it is their decision and hence they will be the ones dealing with the consequences if or when they present themselves. While there is truth behind this reasoning, the consequences of a prescription drug addiction can be extremely extensive. There have been multiple accounts of strong relationships being torn apart, careers derailed, financial situations crippled to the point of homelessness, and lives lost. But these people were not always severe addicts. They used to live a normal life, a life they could call their own. They had dreams, aspirations, goals, all lost to a prescription drug addiction. That is exactly what *The Cork Board* conveys. It illustrates who these people are, the loving relationships they once had, the great lives they enjoyed so very much: not what their addiction transformed them into. In 2017, over 70,000 individuals were killed by a drug overdose. Those people are not just a number; they were someone's friend, significant other, child: they were real people.

Kyle Citrin is a content creator from Madison, Connecticut. At a young age, Kyle pursued his passion for creating cinematic visuals and quickly found success with the national award–winning short The Cork Board. *Throughout his fast-paced lifestyle, his goal is to create stunning visuals and tell memorable stories that evoke emotion.*

Clay Knibbs is a student athlete at Springfield College from Madison, Connecticut. He has witnessed a lot of changes in his life, from sport of choice to overall personality. Clayton himself has had an opioid-related crisis, as one of his direct cousins presumably overdosed on heroin, making this a subject of focus.

Carter Soboleski is a student attending the University of Connecticut, and originally from Madison, Connecticut. He never had any experience working with cameras and editing prior to creating the drug prevention video but has found a love for the art. Carter has also been affected directly by the opioid crisis as he has lost some friends to the crisis.

Climate Change and Prescription Drugs: The Impacts of Increased Temperature on Public Health

Shel Evergreen

I knelt over the garden bed, pruning an overgrown yellow squash on a hot July afternoon, and I felt more sweat on my brow than usual. In Colorado, the summers on the lower-elevation front range are hot and dry. They are much more bearable than the oppressive heat in which I grew up never acclimating to in Oklahoma, but temperatures can still easily reach 100 or degrees or more.

I had recently started taking a selective serotonin reuptake inhibitor to treat complex posttraumatic stress disorder. The benefits had already started to show but so had the side effects: increased sweating, headaches and loss of appetite, among others. I was aware of the side effects and responded to the increased sweating by drinking enough water to ensure hydration and avoid heat exhaustion. But as average temperatures continue to rise and extreme heat events become more frequent, individuals taking medications might face greater impacts to their health.

It can be hard to fully comprehend just how far-reaching the impacts of climate change are, but it touches everything we do, feel, learn and consume. From growing infectious diseases outbreaks to asthmatic attacks due to air pollution, climate change will present an increasingly complex public health dilemma as global temperatures continue to rise.

One of the clearest examples of these public health concerns is the increased risk of heat-related illnesses. Projections show that extreme heat events will become more severe and more frequent in the coming years (Luber and Knowlton 2014). Increased average temperatures, along with an increase in extreme heat events, cause heat exhaustion, heat stroke, and death, especially among vulnerable populations (Portier, et al. 2010).

This increase in extreme heat events will significantly impact those taking certain types of medications. For example, diuretics that are used to treat high blood pressure can cause dehydration, leading to a greater chance of heat exhaustion. Similarly, some allergy medications reduce sweating, which is an important function for cooling the body. And, as I've experienced already, some medications for mental health treatment can lead a person to feel less thirsty or become dehydrated more easily (Pullano 2019).

This issue will likely be experienced in an inequitable way among different populations. Health disparities among vulnerable populations due to climate change have already been documented, and various socioeconomic factors may significantly impact the health of children, older adults, and members of low-income communities and communities of color (Luber and Knowlton 2014). The urban heat island effect is a prime example. "High concentrations of buildings in urban areas cause urban heat island effect, [generating] and absorbing heat, making the urban center several degrees warmer than surrounding areas" (Portier, et al. 2010, 29–31).

These compounding issues may increase the likelihood of certain individuals experiencing heat exhaustion. Imagine a low-income person living in an environment that is more susceptible to the urban heat island effect being prescribed a blood pressure medication. The medical facility is overworked and lacks resources to which more wealthy communities may have access. This person's medical professional then fails to educate the patient that the medication can increase one's risk for heat-related illnesses. The patient must return to work at a construction site outside during the heat of the summer and suffers from heat stroke later that week. Scenarios like this could become more common without adequate preventive measures.

Medical professionals who produce, prescribe, or are otherwise associated with prescription drugs will need to consider the various impacts climate change will have on their dissemination, particularly for vulnerable communities. Some preparedness actions could include education campaigns from public health officials; resources for medical professionals, especially for those working in low-income urban areas; and a commitment from the pharmaceutical industry to incorporate this issue into the planning and production of prescription medications. Further research will also be needed to ensure an effective response, including the understanding of risk factors for illness related to acute and long-term temperature increases, attributes of people who are more resilient to adverse health impacts from heat waves ("Effects of Heat: Climate and Human Health" 2017), and ways to decrease the likelihood of heat-related illnesses for individuals taking prescription medications.

References

"Effects of Heat: Climate and Human Health." 2017. National Institute of Environmental Health Sciences. U.S. Department of Health and Human Services. https://www.niehs.nih.gov/research/programs/geh/climatechange/health_impacts/heat/index.cfm.

Luber, George, and Kim Knowlton. 2014. "Chapter 9: Human Health." In J. M. Melillo, Terese (T.C.) Richmond, and G. W. Yohe, eds. *Climate Change Impacts in the United States: The Third National Climate Assessment*. http://s3.amazonaws.com/nca2014/high/NCA3_Climate_Change_Impacts_in_the_United%20States_HighRes.pdf.

Portier, C. J., et al. 2010. *A Human Health Perspective on Climate Change: A Report Outlining the Research Needs on the Human Health Effects of Climate Change*. Research Triangle Park, NC: Environmental Health Perspectives, National Institute of Environmental Health Sciences.

Pullano, Nina. 2019. "Medications Can Raise Heat Stroke Risk. Are Doctors Prepared to Respond as the Planet Warms?" https://insideclimatenews.org/news/20082019/climate-change-prescription-drug-interaction-heat-stroke-risk-doctors-protocol-research.

Shel Evergreen is a science communication and media professional with a background in energy, climate change, public policy, and equity. Her work philosophy is grounded in solving complex societal challenges through curiosity, creativity, and service to others. One of her favorite quotes is by author and political activist Angela Davis—"You have to act as if it were possible to radically transform the world, and you have to do it all the time."

Drug Discovery: A Twentieth-Century Story of Scientific Curiosity, Persistence, and Creative Guesswork

Margaret Willig Crane

In the late 1950s, the first reports of a radical new treatment for depression reached the United States. Geigy, the Swiss pharmaceutical company, had just launched a drug called imipramine—marketed as Tofranil—in several European countries, and its effects on depressed mood were said to be undeniable.

Until Geigy's discovery, virtually nobody was looking toward a pharmacological solution to the problem of depression. An antidepressant in the form of a pill was simply inconceivable. Depression wasn't understood at the time as a disease with knowable causes, clear symptoms, and a particular pattern or course. Rather, it was seen as an affliction of the human heart, mind, and soul. There was as yet no group of patients suffering from a definable mental illness called depression and hence no market for a drug purporting to treat it.

In 1960, imipramine—the new tricyclic antidepressant (TCA), so-called because of its three-ring molecular structure—was approved in the United States for the treatment of depression, launching a period of discovery in the emerging field of psychopharmacology.

Unexpected Findings

Imipramine was actually discovered by accident during an attempt to improve on the effectiveness of chlorpromazine (Thorazine), the first antipsychotic drug. Its discovery stemmed from an earlier search for drugs to block the destructive action of the hormone histamine.

The early history of psychopharmacological research is fraught with such wrong turns and unintended results. Time after time, a drug developed for the treatment of one condition proved to be far more effective for another. Equally striking is the rapid emergence of drug treatments for mental illness within an extremely short time frame. The TCAs and the monoamine oxidase inhibitors—another class of antidepressants, improbably derived from rocket fuel—came on the scene in the 1950s and early 1960s. These two types of drugs remained the pharmacological treatments of choice for depression until the late 1980s, when Prozac, the first selective serotonin reuptake inhibitor, was approved in the United States. A slew of "me-too" drugs followed, and soon the SSRIs and other new medications rivaled their predecessors for primacy in the clinic and the marketplace.

A Circuitous Path

The story begins in Germany at the height of European industrialization in the late nineteen century. The chemical firm Badische Anilin und Soda Fabrik had manufactured a new series of industrial dyes synthesized from coal tar, including one called methylene blue. In 1883, a chemist named August Bernthsen analyzed the chemical structure of methylene blue and used his insights to develop the first phenothiazine compound. That compound, and dozens of others in the same series, languished for the next sixty years, when the trail was picked up in France.

During the 1930s, French researchers began a focused search for an agent capable of countering the effects of histamine. At the time, this hormone was believed to trigger "stress" and "shock"—terms that connoted the collapse of the cardiovascular system in response to blood loss or serious infection, especially in the aftermath of surgery. The need for an effective antihistamine was perceived as urgent. Rising to the challenge, the Pasteur Institute collaborated with the laboratories of Rhône-Poulenc to develop phenbenzamine (Antergan) and diphenhydramine (Benadryl), still used today by people the world over to prevent and control allergic reactions.

The twists and turns leading from a chemically distinct industrial dye to modern antihistamines and antidepressants appear random at first glance. The missing piece that completes the puzzle is the curiosity of generations of scientists following their hunches. That curiosity, along with persistence and creative insight, was ultimately responsible for connecting these seemingly far-flung discoveries. Along the way, these investigators tolerated failure after failure before they obtained positive results.

Basic versus Clinical Research

In earlier times, drug discovery was weighted toward basic or *pure* research, defined as follows in a 1953 report by the National Science Foundation: "Basic research is performed without thought of practical ends. . . . The scientist doing basic research may not be at all interested in the practical applications of his work, yet the further progress of industrial development would eventually stagnate if basic research were long neglected" (What Is Basic Research 1953, 88).

In the latter decades of the twentieth century, however, basic research—the underpinning of drug discovery—began to be folded into *research and development*, or R&D. Today's basic research often takes a backseat to translational research, which aims to build on basic research findings to create new therapies, medical procedures, or diagnostics, and clinical research—the testing of new medications, devices, and diagnostics for safety and effectiveness, at first in animals and then in humans.

Like any business, the modern pharmaceutical industry is driven by the need to be profitable. Private industry is not designed to support the open-ended, trial-and-error-based efforts of the pure-research scientist.

With the advent of twenty-first-century high-throughput technology, genetics and genomics, and cell-based therapeutics, basic research has become more "rational" than in days gone by. And yet the intuitive insights of basic science researchers, and their willingness to take risks based on a hunch, will always be part of the mix, as creative "failures" lead to tomorrow's breakthroughs.

Urgent Need

Nowhere are breakthroughs more urgently needed than in the class of drugs called anti-infectives, also known as antibiotics. The rise of antibiotic-resistant tuberculosis worldwide and the emergence of drug-resistant "superbugs," such as methicillin-resistant *Staphylococcus aureus*, the culprit in many hospital-borne infections, exemplify the sense of urgency surrounding the need for new antibiotics that go beyond the me-too paradigm, which privileges the development of drugs that are substantially similar to those already on the market.

Overall, antibiotics have been unprofitable for the pharmaceutical industry, which suggests that the federal government may need to step in to fund all three types of research—basic, translational, and clinical—to stem the tide of resistance to the antibiotics currently used, and often overused, to fight deadly infectious diseases.

Margaret Willig Crane is a freelance health and medical writer based in New York City. Her work has appeared in The Scientist, *in the* Los Angeles Times, *and on numerous health and educational websites.*

Will Naloxone Become a Real "Superhero"?

Randolph Fillmore

The National Institute on Drug Abuse (NIDA) website poses a big question: *How Did This Happen?* (National Institute on Drug Abuse 2020a).

The question refers to the addiction and overdose problem with opioids, a class of drugs that include hydrocodone and oxycontin developed and marketed to fight serious pain. The drugs work well, but they have also led to an epidemic of addiction and death for many who overdose on them.

While some answers to the question have been unraveled, a better question now might be, *How Do We Fix This?*

Some answers to this question can be found on the National Institutes of Health (NIH) website; the NIH places lots of life-saving hope on a drug called naloxone (National Institutes of Health 2020).

Naloxone is also an opioid, but it is an antagonist, or "enemy," to other opioids. When an opioid overdose causes respiratory suppression and potential breathing cessation, an injection of naloxone can reverse the effects of opioid overdose, restore breathing, and save a life—if it is administered in time.

While naloxone has been saving lives for years, the NIDA website, which tracks opioid overdose deaths state by state, still offers a bleak scenario, showing that, even with the availability of naloxone expanding, opioid overdose deaths continue to be a national problem. States such as Ohio, West Virginia, Maryland, New Hampshire, Massachusetts, and the District of Columbia (Washington, D.C.), despite the benefit of naloxone, lead the nation, averaging twenty-eight opioid overdose deaths per 100,000 residents (National Institute on Drug Abuse 2018).

The use of injectable naloxone has been restricted to first responders and medical professionals. However, the U.S.

Department of Health and Human Services (HHS) and the NIH are copromoting increased and more open and timely access to naloxone (National Institute on Drug Abuse 2020b). Efforts to make the drug available in pharmacies, with or without a prescription, are also gaining support.

Naloxone Access Expanding

"The overdose-reversing drug naloxone saves lives—but only if it's readily available when an overdose occurs," said the Centers for Disease Control and Prevention (CDC) in an August 2019 statement ("Still Not Enough Naloxone Where It's Most Needed" 2019). CDC's "key findings" include the following:

- The number of naloxone prescriptions dispensed doubled from 2017 to 2018.
- Only one naloxone prescription is dispensed for every seventy high-dose opioid prescriptions nationwide.
- Most (71%) Medicare prescriptions for naloxone required a copay, compared to 42% for commercial insurance.
- Rural counties were nearly three times more likely to be a low-dispensing county compared to metropolitan counties.
- Naloxone dispensing is twenty-five times greater in the highest-dispensing counties than the lowest-dispensing counties. (Centers for Disease Control and Prevention 2020).

According to the CDC, "too few doctors are prescribing naloxone to patients receiving high-dose opioids or opioids plus benzodiazepines, or to those with a substance use disorder, as recommended by CDC's Guideline for Prescribing Opioids for Chronic Pain. Nearly one million more naloxone prescriptions could have been dispensed in 2018 if every patient with a high-dose opioid prescription were offered naloxone" (Centers for Disease Control and Prevention 2019).

CDC also says that up-to-date information on pharmacy-based naloxone dispensing is needed and that the agency is examining how naloxone is dispensed from U.S. retail pharmacies at the national and county levels and advocating change to make it more available.

While the CDC's findings show an increase in naloxone pharmacy dispensing between 2012 and 2018, study data confirm that additional efforts are needed to improve naloxone access at the local level as wide regional variations in dispensing in pharmacies exist, despite consistent state laws.

For example, in 2018, rural counties in the United States had the lowest naloxone dispensing rates. Additionally, primary care providers wrote only 1.5 naloxone prescriptions per 100 high-dose opioid prescriptions—a marker for opioid overdose risk—and over half of naloxone prescriptions required a copay.

The Pharmacy Connection

Recent pharmacy dispensing statistics are encouraging, however. A 2017 study by the National Bureau of Economic Research found that "the adoption of naloxone is associated with a nine percent decrease in opioid-related deaths not involving heroin. . . . Our results suggest that removing criminal liability for possession of naloxone is an important feature of these laws. Removing criminal liability for possession of naloxone is associated with a 13 percent reduction in opioid-related deaths" (Rees, et al. 2017).

Many states now allow *third party* and *standing orders* for naloxone distribution. Third-party prescribing allows a prescriber to write a prescription for a medication to someone other than the intended user of the medication. A standing order is a mechanism by which a health care provider with prescribing privileges, including a state health officer, writes a prescription that covers a large group of people. Not all states permit both mechanisms (American Medical Association 2020).

There have also been calls for naloxone to be co-prescribed along with opioids, so people have it on hand if needed. In 2017, an American Medical Association Opioid Task Force encouraged physicians to consider co-prescribing naloxone when it is clinically appropriate to do so. The task force added that this should be a decision to be made primarily between the patient and the physician and that "factors" may be helpful in determining whether to co-prescribe naloxone to a patient, to a family member, or to a close friend of the patient (Safe Project 2020).

Naloxone News

In late 2015, the U.S. Food and Drug Administration (FDA) approved a nasal spray device for naloxone administration. That was a big step toward making naloxone both more available and easier to use (National Institute on Drug Abuse 2015).

"This easy-to-use intranasal formulation will no doubt save many lives," said Nora Volkow, managing director of the NIDA in a 2015 FDA press release.

Fast forward to 2020: another big step was the FDA's approval of new labeling that helps clear naloxone to be available over the counter, which means naloxone could be available without a prescription. To make this change, the FDA studied 710 adults, some of whom were opioid users, to determine if they understood the labeling directions well enough to use naloxone safely, when and where needed. The study, which concluded that its participants could understand the directions, was published in the *New England Journal of Medicine* in late June 2020 ("FDA Labeling Study Helps Clear Path for OTC Naloxone" 2020).

Conclusion

Most experts agree that the opioid overdose rates and resulting deaths are declining but that the problem will not be overcome until there are new, nonaddictive drugs to fight serious pain.

Having an effective pain reliever that does not lead to dependency would be a pharmaceutical *holy grail*, according to Andrew Coop, a professor at the University of Maryland Baltimore School of Pharmacy: "We need a drug for which there

is no reinforcement, one that does not have an abuse liability."
Coop says he and colleagues are working on developing just
such a drug (Fillmore 2018).

References

American Medical Association. 2020. "End the Epidemic."
   https://www.end-opioid-epidemic.org/naloxone/.

Centers for Disease Control and Prevention. 2019. "Opioid
   'Key Findings.'" https://www.cdc.gov/media/releases/2019/
   p0806-naloxone.html.

Centers for Disease Control and Prevention. 2020. "Opioid
   Overdose." https://www.cdc.gov/drugoverdose/.

"FDA Labeling Study Helps Clear Path for OTC Naloxone."
   2020. Regulatory Focus. https://www.raps.org/news-
   and-articles/news-articles/2020/5/fda-labeling-study-
   helps-clear-path-for-otc-naloxo.

Fillmore, Randolph. 2018 "Opioid Crisis Sparks Action."
   University of Maryland School of Pharmacy Magazine.
   https://issuu.com/umbsop/docs/capsule-winter2018final.

National Institute on Drug Abuse. 2015. "FDA Approves
   Naloxone Nasal Spray." https://archives.drugabuse.gov/
   news-events/news-releases/2015/11/fda-approves-naloxone-
   nasal-spray-to-reverse-opioid-overdose.

National Institute on Drug Abuse. 2020a. "Opioid Overdose
   Crisis—How Did This Happen?" https://www.drugabuse
   .gov/drug-topics/opioids/opioid-overdose-crisis.

National Institute on Drug Abuse. 2020b. "Opioid Overdose
   Reversal with Naloxone (Narcan, Evzio) NIH Naloxone."
   https://www.drugabuse.gov/drug-topics/opioids/
   opioid-overdose-reversal-naloxone-narcan-evzio.

National Institute on Drug Abuse. 2018. "Opioid Summaries
   by State." https://www.drugabuse.gov/drug-topics/opioids/
   opioid-summaries-by-state.

National Institutes of Health. 2020. "HEAL Initiative Research Plan." https://heal.nih.gov/about/research-plan.

Rees, Daniel I., et al. 2017. "With a Little Help from My Friends: The Effects of Naloxone Access and Good Samaritan Laws on Opioid-Related Deaths." National Bureau of Economic Research. https://www.nber.org/papers/w23171.pdf.

Safe Project. 2020. "State Naloxone Access Rules and Resources." https://www.safeproject.us/naloxone-awareness-project/state-rules/.

"Still Not Enough Naloxone Where It's Most Needed." 2019. Centers for Disease Control and Prevention. https://www.cdc.gov/media/releases/2019/p0806-naloxone.html.

Randolph Fillmore is the director of Florida Science Communications, Inc.

Drugs and the Professional Bodybuilder

Kenzie Gauck

When you think of bodybuilding, I'm sure the big names come to mind: Arnold Schwarzenegger, Lou Ferrigno, Ronnie Coleman, and so forth. But bodybuilding has gained a larger following since then and is now becoming a popular sport. The sport of bodybuilding has grown so much so that there are multiple conventions held throughout the year where people from all over the world compete: events like TheFitExpo, Arnold Sports Festival, and Olympia Fitness & Performance Weekend. But where did it all start and how do these competitors get so big? And what does this have to do with prescription drugs?

Bodybuilding's history cannot be pinned down to an exact date, however; the first ever bodybuilding competition was held in 1891. Back when this show debuted, the form bodybuilding took was much different to the one it has now. Now, those who compete have otherworldly body proportions and physiques, and these body types have become the golden standard to which all serious bodybuilders compare themselves. The 1940s and 1950s saw an uptick in this type of physique, but it wasn't until the 1970s when "the muscular body became more desirable, the gym industry gained momentum, and the industry as a whole became lucrative" (Robson 2019). Here is where you see large, muscular men, like Arnold, competing on stage for largest muscle mass and, in order to beat these types of competitors, you had to be bigger than the next guy.

So how do you get to be so big? Surely, it's more complicated than just going to the gym and having a balanced diet. Well, in a way, you'd be right. Yes, there are plenty of bodybuilders out there who do not desire to compete with the behemoths on stage and they just do it because they like the look. These people can achieve a very muscular physique with just consistent gym exercise and a strict diet, but if you want to be on stage and actually be competitive, you will find that a lot of them look for outside help. Bodybuilders will often turn to pharmacological assistance and use drugs like insulin, human growth hormone, and/or anabolic steroids in order to "enhance muscle hypertrophy, speed recovery and prevent the effects of overtraining, increase training intensity and aggressiveness, control fat, body water, and appetite" (Fahey 1997, 145). Some of these drugs are used on their own or in combination with others in order to achieve whatever desired effect the user is after. For instance, a bodybuilder who wants to "feed muscles during intense exercise, prevent muscle breakdown, and help [with] performance" might inject himself with insulin (DeNoon 2003) and/or use anabolic steroids to gain weight and increase muscle size and strength. Human growth hormone acts in the same way as anabolic steroids in that it is used to increase muscle mass, but it is naturally produced by the pituitary gland, unlike steroids, which are synthetically created.

As you might assume, these particular pharmaceuticals are not available over the counter and are generally not prescribed without good reason. So how and where from do they get them? In some cases, you can get legitimate prescriptions from a doctor if there is a medical need. However, bodybuilding is not seen as a medical need. For example, testosterone injections are popularly used by bodybuilders to gain muscle mass and endurance and can be easily acquired with a prescription. However, testosterone is usually prescribed only in males with low levels of testosterone, generally middle-aged men. If a young man in his 20s to 30s sees a doctor asking for a testosterone prescription, he might as well not waste his time because odds are he won't be getting one. This is why most bodybuilders turn to Internet pharmacies to get what they need. Oftentimes, these Internet pharmacies are overseas and do not have to adhere to FDA standards and regulations in order to sell their products. Users take them at their own risk—of which there are many.

The risks associated with anabolic steroids can vary from men to women, with side effects ranging from prominent breasts, infertility, and shrunken testicles in men to a deeper voice, baldness, and increased body hair in women. More severe risks include liver abnormalities and tumors, high blood pressure, psychiatric disorders, and heart and blood circulation problems, while the risks associated with human growth hormone have ranged from vision problems, joint pain, an enlarged heart, and high blood pressure (Mayo Clinic 2019). These risks, to a lot of bodybuilders, are worth the sacrifice in order to obtain their peak physique, and there are many bodybuilders out there who only take these types of performance enhancers and never feeling the need to touch insulin. I've been around bodybuilders of many competitive levels and by and large, what I have seen is that most won't touch insulin. Why is that? Plainly because it has more risks associated with it, chief among them being hypoglycemic comas, which can potentially lead to death.

There is no denying that these performance enhancers work; otherwise, they wouldn't be so universally used, and there is obviously a large market for these kinds of medications, but there is often little to no formal user education on what these drugs can potentially do. It's one thing if these steroids were obtained legally, through a physician, for an actual medical condition, but another thing entirely when they are acquired illegally and with no formal education on how to use them. There are millions of people who use insulin and testosterone on a daily basis, but they use it for its intended purposes. When you start using a drug for off-label uses, you may get your desired outcome, but at what cost?

References

DeNoon, Daniel J. 2003. "Insulin for Bodybuilding Can Kill." WebMD. www.webmd.com/fitness-exercise/ news/20030804/insulin-for-bodybuilding-can-kill.

Fahey, Thomas D. 1997. "Pharmacology of Bodybuiling." In T. Reilly and M. Orme, eds. *The Clinical Pharmacology of Sports and Exercise.* http://esteve.org/wp-content/ uploads/2018/01/138346.pdf.

Mayo Clinic. 2019. "Understanding the Risks of Performance-Enhancing Drugs." www .mayoclinic.org/healthy-lifestyle/fitness/in-depth/ performance-enhancing-drugs/art-20046134.

Robson, David. 2019. "A History Lesson in Bodybuilding." Bodybuilding.com. www.bodybuilding.com/fun/ drobson61.htm.

Kenzie Gauck has over ten years of experience in the medical field ranging from environmental work to pharmacology, to autoimmune research. She has been published on PLOS One *for her work in the autoimmune field. She currently resides in Cincinnati, Ohio, with her fiancé and two dogs.*

The Significance of Statistics

Joel Grossman

Ronald Aylmer Fisher's "statistical significance" tests and theories of randomization and experimental design for "controlled experiments" are scientific pillars for prescription drug and vaccine approval. Medical innovations traditionally arose from observation and "uncontrolled experiments" or trial and error. "Keen observation" in 1796 led Edward Jenner to conduct "uncontrolled experiments" inoculating harmless cowpox virus into skin wounds to protect against the deadly smallpox virus (Fisher 1951). Once England's king and queen consented to be experimental subjects and survived, the whole nation joined the vaccination bandwagon. Today, rather than immediate adoption, Jenner's observations would be starting point for several years of phased testing (controlled experiments) for safety (Phase I), dosage (Phase II), and efficacy (Phase III).

Controlled experiments use statistics to compare drug effects with no treatment, placebo, or other therapies. "Need for control arises from the experimenter's consciousness that he is ignorant of innumerable causes which may affect his experimental results," wrote Fisher (1951). "It was for this reason that controlled experimentation was first developed and refined" in the early twentieth century.

"Each case came to him as a unique problem" at Rothamsted Agricultural Experiment Station, wrote Fisher's statistician daughter, Joan Fisher Box (1978). "There was not in those days a wide repertoire of statistical methods on which he could draw," so "he had to be inventive and ingenious. . . . Later he was to deplore how often his own methods were applied thoughtlessly, as cookbook solutions, when they were inappropriate." Statistical significance tests were never intended to displace other evidence, context, details behind the raw data, and so forth.

"Fisher is the undisputed creator of the modern field that statisticians call the design of experiments," wrote Leonard Savage (1976) in *The Annals of Statistics*. "He preached effectively against the maxim of varying one factor at a time" and "taught how to make many comparisons" in one experiment. "The analysis of variance and the analysis of covariance are his terms." Randomized design also "seems to have originated with Fisher . . . though this technique is so fundamental to modern statistics that to credit Fisher with it sounds like attributing the invention of the wheel to Mr. So and So."

For Rothamsted's food crop experiments, Fisher "presumed" the laws of chance were operative with "Nature" randomizing weather conditions within the prevailing climate. In controlled drug experiments, researchers supply randomization to eliminate inadvertent bias. In double blind experiments, neither researchers nor patients know who is getting the drug. "The only modification of the art of experimentation, as developed on statistical principles, which does not flow directly from the requirement to maximize the amount of information, obtainable with limited resources, consists in the introduction into the experimental procedure of what is called randomization," wrote Fisher (1947). "Without it our tests of significance would be worthless."

"It was in the study of experimental data that the characteristics of modern statistics first began to display themselves, notably in that series of methods which are known as the tests of significance," wrote Fisher (1951). "The logical situation behind these is exceedingly simple, though it has been seriously obscured in recent times by the elaboration of a highly sophisticated mathematical background. This, however, is unnecessary."

In 1909, William Sealy Gosset, a Guinness beer brewer consulting Fisher, developed the "Student's t-test," the "first clearly exemplified" test of statistical significance, to compare yeast and barley varieties. Guinness employees were forbidden from publishing after a master brewer exposed trade secrets. So Gosset wrote at night at home and clandestinely published under the name "Student." But Fisher "developed most of the significance testing methods now in general use," wrote David Salsburg (2001), the first statistician hired by Big Pharma (Pfizer). Fisher "referred to the probability that allows one to declare significance as the 'p-value'" but "never indicates exactly what p-value one might call significant."

Flip open a medical or scientific journal reporting experiments. At the bottom of a table of numbers labeled "Results" is a "statistical significance" shorthand notation: usually "($p < 0.05$)." This p-value is a branding of sorts, like a seal of approval, telling readers that repeating the experiment 100 times yields different results 5% (0.05; or 1 in 20) of the time. Thus "$p < 0.05$" is "95% significance" (0.95; or 19 in 20), the gold standard for prescription drug approval. However, *95% significance* was never intended to preclude other clinical evidence or be dogma chiseled in stone and slavishly obeyed. Indeed, 99% ($p < 0.01$) and 80% ($p < 0.20$) are also valid.

Even seasoned medical professionals experience difficulty evaluating controlled drug experiments and marketing literature claiming statistical significance. An experimental design for an antibiotic ointment applied to sutured wounds was mind bogglingly described in the *British Medical Journal* (*BMJ*) as a "randomised placebo controlled double blind superiority trial." It was presented as a "statistical question" to show doctors that prescription drugs can be marketed as providing statistically significant (95%) results yet be practically worthless (Sedgwick 2014).

"Clinical significance cannot necessarily be inferred from statistical significance, and statistical significance cannot be inferred from clinical significance," though the terms are often used interchangeably, wrote Sedgwick (2014). A third term, *patient significance*, best describes whether cost and compliance sufficiently benefit patients.

Researchers can manipulate and reverse engineer experimental designs to recruit the "right number" of patients to achieve 95% statistical significance ($p < 0.05$). Call it conjuring a marketing mountain out of a molehill: making a drug of minimal value falsely appear clinically significant. In the *BMJ* antibiotic experiment, a sufficiently large sample size, 473 patients per group, produced statistical significance ($p < 0.05$): 11 percent less wound infection with ointment; 6.6 percent with placebo. But the 4.4 percent benefit justified neither drug cost nor patient inconvenience. "In effect, the trial was overpowered" to produce statistical significance, wrote Sedgwick (2014). With under 473 patients per treatment group, no significant drug effect was detectable.

In a *BMJ* "Medicine and History" article on Fisher and statistics, Cyril Clarke (1990) mentioned a more subjective, gut-level significance test:

> "If it's significant it hits you in the eye; if it doesn't it isn't." This was spoken by a distinguished surgeon and has cheered up multitudes of hard working clinicians, suggesting to them that they need not after all understand the intricacies of statistical language.

Underpowered experiments (too few patients) are typical for rare diseases like Duchenne muscular dystrophy (DMD), making it mathematically difficult to achieve 95% significance and gain new drug approval. A muscular degeneration linked to X-chromosome genes, DMD afflicts 1 in 5,000 young males, who lose walking ability by their mid-teens and die young. "As I can assure you from personal experience in caring for such patients, words cannot adequately express either the heartbreak of the parents of DMD patients or the suffering patiently endured by those who are afflicted by this terrible ailment," wrote Stein (2016).

Eteplirsen, a drug targeting 13 percent of patients with DMD with the "exon 51" genetic defect, restored walking ability in six-minute walking tests with 99% significance ($p < 0.01$) with no adverse effects in eleven patients: in other words, high *patient significance* and *clinical significance* in an "underpowered" experiment. But a U.S. Food and Drug Administration (FDA) panel of outside scientific experts instead focused on a biochemical marker, the muscle protein dystrophin, which was not significantly elevated.

"You might think this story would quickly end happily—for patients, for their parents, and for the doctors who treat DMD—as a joyful FDA overwhelmingly approved" the drug, wrote Stein (2016). "Despite a 'legion' of eteplirsen advocates—including over 100 members of Congress—an FDA advisory panel, by a 6–7 vote, wasn't convinced." The expert panel recommended a decade of basic research and $400 million for larger experiments (more patients) to "tease out" statistical significance.

Besides too few patients on planet Earth with the genetic defect for large, "overpowered" experiments, the small drug company faced bankruptcy without drug approval. Top FDA officials, realizing this was a life-threatening disease with no alternatives, overruled their scientific panel and approved eteplirsen. Scientific experts exploded into public outrage. *Forbes* magazine called it a "civil war" within the FDA (Herper 2016). But now multiple drugs targeting other DMD genes are being developed worldwide. Thus, clinical significance and patient significance are valid alternatives to statistical significance.

References

Box, Joan Fisher. 1978. *RA Fisher: The Life of a Scientist*. New York: Wiley.

Clarke, Cyril. 1990. "Professor Sir Ronald Fisher, FRS." *British Medical Journal*. 301(6766):1446. https://www

.ncbi.nlm.nih.gov/pmc/articles/PMC1679832/pdf/
bmj00211-0050.pdf.

Fisher, Ronald Aylmer. 1947. "Development of the Theory
of Experimental Design." *Proceedings of the International
Statistical Conferences.* 3:434–439. http://hdl.handle
.net/2440/15254.

Fisher, Ronald Aylmer. 1951. *Statistics. In Scientific Thought in
the Twentieth Century.* London: Watts. http://hdl.handle
.net/2440/15261.

Herper, Matthew. 2016. "Approving a Muscular Dystrophy
Drug Ignites a Civil War at the FDA." *Forbes.* https://www
.forbes.com/sites/matthewherper/2016/09/20/approving-
a-muscular-dystrophy-drug-ignites-civil-war-at-the-
fda/#757dfc0b72a8.

Salsburg, David. 2001. *The Lady Tasting Tea.* New York:
Henry Holt.

Savage, Leonard J. 1976. "On Rereading RA Fisher." *The
Annals of Statistics.* 4(3): 441–500. https://projecteuclid
.org/download/pdf_1/euclid.aos/1176343456.

Sedgwick, Philip. 2014. "Clinical Significance versus Statistical
Significance." *BMJ Online* 348. https://www.researchgate
.net/profile/Philip_Sedgwick/publication/275073947_
Clinical_significance_versus_statistical_significance/
links/56e7f6c008ae9aecadbaac72.pdf.

Stein, Cy A. 2016. "Eteplirsen Approved for Duchenne
Muscular Dystrophy: The FDA Faces a Difficult Choice."
Molecular Therapy. 24(11): 1884–1885. https://www.cell
.com/molecular-therapy-family/molecular-therapy/pdf/
S1525-0016(16)45439-0.pdf.

Joel Grossman began reading The Lady Tasting Tea *to understand why 98 percent of the 2016 U.S. presidential election polls
were proved wrong. He writes the Biocontrol Beat blog.*

Prescription Drug Ads That Target Consumers

Phill Jones

The marketing of prescription drugs directly to consumers fuels controversy. The United States is one of only two countries that allow the practice of direct-to-consumer (DTC) advertising of prescription drugs, the other being New Zealand.

The Development of DTC Marketing

At one time, pharmaceutical companies decided if a drug should be sold over the counter or by prescription. In 1951, the U.S. Congress passed legislation that created a definition of prescription drugs to include drugs that are not safe to use except under the supervision of a practitioner licensed to administer the drugs. The new rule attempted to protect consumers from self-administering potentially harmful drugs.

If a drug were only available by a doctor's prescription, the company that manufactured the drug targeted advertising of the drug at health professionals. By the 1960s, drug companies focused promotions on doctors, pharmacists, and hospitals. The U.S. Food and Drug Administration (FDA 2015) regulated prescription drug advertising, requiring that ads must not be false or misleading, must present both risks and benefits of a drug, and must include a summary of known risks.

During the 1970s, a patients' rights movement coupled with patients' increasing concerns about prescription drug use led to consumers' demand for information about these drugs (Donahue 2006). A few pharmaceutical companies responded to this demand by offering drug information directly to the public. In 1985, the FDA decided to allow DTC marketing of prescription drugs on the condition that the ads met the same legal requirements as those targeted at physicians. That is, a drug ad would have to include a statement about side effects, effectiveness, and circumstances in which the drug should not be used.

Although this type of information could be included—in small print—for newspaper and magazine ads, the requirement was impractical for broadcast ads.

Bowing to pressure, the FDA eased the data requirement for broadcast advertisements in 1997. Drug companies could refer consumers to various sources for detailed information about a drug, including websites and toll-free phone numbers. The change in advertising rules opened a floodgate for DTC marketing. Investments in consumer-targeted prescription drug ads surged from $1.3 billion in 1997 to $6 billion by 2016 (Schwartz and Woloshin 2019). DTC ads flourished on TV. According to one report, more than 770,000 TV drug ads were broadcast during 2016 (Kaufman 2017). DTC advertisements also emerged on social networks, such as Facebook.

The Controversy of DTC Prescription Drug Marketing

Proponents of DTC marketing argue that advertisements educate the public about the marketed drug and health conditions that the drug is intended to treat. For example, PhRMA, the Pharmaceutical Research and Manufacturers of America, has asserted that DTC ads for prescription drugs increase awareness of diseases, inform consumers about treatment options, motivate consumers to discuss health concerns with their physicians, and encourage patients to comply with prescription drug treatment procedures (PhRMA 2018).

During a 2002 interview for *Frontline*, Sidney Taurel, then chairman, president, and CEO of pharmaceutical company Eli Lilly, stated that DTC advertising offers important public health benefits (Taurel 2002). He said that the majority of advertised products are intended to treat conditions that are undertreated, such as high cholesterol and hypertension and that DTC ads educate consumers about these conditions, which encourages discussions with doctors.

Some, however, fail to see the benefits of DTC marketing. During November 2004, the FDA released the results of a 500-physician survey about the effects of DTC prescription drug promotion on patient-doctor relationships (FDA 2015). Doctors thought that prescription drug ads failed to convey information about the risks and benefits equally well. About 75 percent of the doctors said that the ads caused patients to believe that a drug is more effective than it is in practice. Many doctors felt pressure to prescribe an advertised drug.

Yale University researchers reviewed DTC TV ads for prescription drugs aired in the United States between January 2015 and July 2016. Their findings suggested that the information provided in the advertisements is unreliable and potentially misleading. "The promotion of off-label indications [i.e., unapproved uses], poor quality of information, distracting risk presentations, and the fact that risks are never quantified could distort the perception of benefit and risk information," they said (Klara, Kim, and Ross 2018).

Investigative health reporter Martha Rosenberg offered a less restrained criticism of DTC prescription drug marketing. "DTC advertising has done two pernicious things," she said. "It has created a nation of hypochondriacs with depression, bipolar disorder, GERD [gastroesophageal reflux disease], Restless Legs, insomnia, seasonal allergies and assorted pain, mood and 'risk' conditions and it has reduced doctors to order takers and gate keepers" (Rosenberg 2014; italics in the original).

Professor Richard L. Kravitz and his colleagues contributed to the debate about the advantages and disadvantages of DTC prescription drug advertising. "Proponents argue that it serves an educational mission," they said. "Others argue that it is contradictory to have a category of drugs called 'prescription,' made available through those with specialized training, yet allow those same drugs to be marketed to persons who lack that specialized knowledge" (Wilkes, Bell, and Kravitz 2000).

Searching for a Resolution to the DTC Ad Controversy

In 2015, the American Medical Association proposed a way to terminate the DTC ad controversy: a ban on DTC ads of prescription drugs. This simple solution, however, probably would not survive litigation. Judges have considered advertising to be a form of "commercial speech," and they have ruled that a ban on advertising violates First Amendment protections of freedom of speech.

To improve the educational quality of DTC prescription drug ads, PhRMA issued guiding principles for such ads in 2005 and 2008. Researchers reviewed ads broadcast on U.S. television during 2016 (Applequist and Ball 2018). They concluded that self-regulation had little effect; drugs continued to promote products above educating the public.

Another approach for improving the quality of DTC drug ads would be to require the FDA to approve ads before they were made available to the public. The FDA could ensure that an advertisement includes appropriate risk warnings and educational content, and the agency could impose sanctions for misleading claims (Foley and Gross 2000). Congress would have to grant this authority to the FDA. As of early 2021, no such actions have occurred.

References

Applequist, J., and J. G. Ball. 2018. "An Updated Analysis of Direct-to-Consumer Television Advertisements for Prescription Drugs." *Annals of Family Medicine*. 16(3): 211–216.

Donahue, J. 2006. "A History of Drug Advertising: The Evolving Roles of Consumers and Consumer Protection." *The Milbank Quarterly*. 84(4): 659–699.

FDA. 2015. "The Impact of Direct-to-Consumer Advertising." https://www.fda.gov/drugs/drug-infor mation-consumers/impact-direct-consumer-advertising.

Foley, L. and D. Gross. 2000. "In Brief: Are Consumers Well Informed about Prescription Drugs? The Impact of Printed Direct-to-Consumer Advertising." https://www.aarp.org/ health/drugs-supplements/info-04-2000/aresearch-import-15-INB15.html.

Kaufman, J. 2017. "Think You're Seeing More Drug Ads on TV? You Are, and Here's Why." https://www.nytimes .com/2017/12/24/business/media/prescription-drugs- advertising-tv.html.

Klara, K., J. Kim, and J. S. Ross. 2018. "Direct-to-Consumer Broadcast Advertisements for Pharmaceuticals: Off-Label Promotion and Adherence to FDA Guidelines." *JGIM: Journal of General Internal Medicine*. 33(5): 651–658.

PhRMA. 2018. "PhRMA Guiding Principles: Direct to Consumer Advertisements About Prescription Medicines." https://www.phrma.org/codes-and-guidelines/ direct-to-consumer-advertising-principles.

Rosenberg, M. 2014. "Following Success of DTC Drug Advertising, DTC Radiation Advertising? What?" https:// www.centerforhealthjournalism.org/2014/02/13/following- success-dtc-drug-advertising-dtc-radiation-advertising-what.

Schwartz, L.M. and S. Woloshin. 2019. "Medical Marketing in the United States, 1997–2016." *JAMA*. 32(1)1: 80–96.

Taurel, S. 2002. "Interview: Sidney Taurel." https://www.pbs .org/wgbh/pages/frontline/shows/other/interviews/taurel .html.

Wilkes, M.S., R.A. Bell, and R.L. Kravitz. 2000. "Direct-To- Consumer Prescription Drug Advertising: Trends, Impact, and Implications." *Health Affairs*. 19(2): 110–128.

Phillip Jones, PhD, JD, writes articles and books in the areas of general science, agricultural biotechnology, forensic science, medicine, history, and law.

The Human Brain

Maia Pujara

Every day, your brain pumps out its very own concoction of drugs, or chemicals. These chemicals control everything, from making you fall asleep to making you fall in love.

Just like how the skin is made up of skin cells, the brain is made up of tiny cells called neurons. Neurons are special because, unlike skin cells, they talk to each other very fast using electrical and chemical signals. The chemicals that your brain makes are called neurotransmitters. The neurotransmitters attach themselves to special places on the neuron called receptors to get their message across.

Think of a neurotransmitter as a text message that one neuron sends to another neuron and the receptor as the cell phone. And let's say our friend Katie is sleepy. In Katie's brain, neuron 1 sends a "text"—a neurotransmitter molecule—from its cell phone to neuron 2's cell phone saying, "Hey, neuron 2, you might want to tell Katie to turn off her phone so she can close her eyes and fall asleep." And then, thousands upon thousands of Katie's other neurons send each other neurotransmitter "texts" back and forth on their cell phones, so she can shut off her phone, close her eyes, and finally fall asleep.

Your brain is made up of about one hundred billion neurons. This means a lot of neurotransmitter "text messages" are happening at once to keep things running smoothly.

Prescription Drugs: How Exactly Do They Work in the Brain?

Prescription drugs are chemicals designed to work with the brain's natural chemistry—in fact, they look and act very similar to the chemicals in the brain. Though these drugs can help people feel better, they're not perfect. There is no "miracle" drug. There can be surprising side effects because of how they work in the brain, and addiction can happen if someone takes a drug for longer than needed.

Sleep Drugs: GABA

When you fall asleep, your brain activity decreases because of a neurotransmitter called gamma aminobutyric acid, or GABA, for short. Now let's say Katie has been having problems falling asleep no matter what she tries. Her doctor prescribes a drug for a sleep disorder called insomnia, an inability to fall asleep. Because this drug helps neurons release more GABA, Katie is able to fall asleep very well at night. Sadly, she also starts getting headaches, muscle aches, sleepier during the day, scatter-brained, and dizzy (National Institute on Drug Abuse 2015). Katie's doctor also warned her that, because the drug is so strong, it could be deadly when combined with other drugs such as cold medicine, alcohol, or painkillers. All of those drugs also work on GABA receptors and slow down brain activity, heart rate, and breathing.

Painkillers: Opioids

Let's say Katie oversleeps and is late to class. Panicking and rushing out of bed, she trips, falls, and breaks her ankle. In Katie's brain, neurons are talking—no, yelling and screaming—to each other about how painful a broken bone feels. There are natural neurotransmitters called opioids attaching themselves to opioid receptors on neurons to dial down the pain, but this is not enough. So Katie's doctor prescribes her painkillers, which are stronger opioids. Although opioids are good at bringing down moderate to severe pain, they can make a person feel drowsy, confused, nauseous, constipated, and short of breath (National Institute on Drug Abuse 2014).

Stimulants: Dopamine and Norepinephrine

With everything Katie has been dealing with, she can no longer pay attention in class. She goes to a doctor who prescribes her a drug that will help her focus her attention. This type of drug, called a stimulant, helps neurons release natural neurotransmitters called dopamine and norepinephrine. Dopamine is important for motivating movements and for feeling good, while norepinephrine helps us pay attention and focus. Just like the other drugs, stimulants help improve attention and focus but can come with some nasty side effects, including chest pains, stomachaches, and feelings of fear or anger. If they are taken for too long, they can cause deadly seizures and irregular heartbeats (National Institute on Drug Abuse 2015).

Long-Term Effects on the Brain and Addiction

The brain is wired such that, if it comes across something that feels good, it will continue to look for that special something, to bring that feeling back again (Bragdon and Gamon 2000, 28). Prescription drugs, especially painkillers and stimulants, can be addictive because they can make a person feel very good.

Although all of the different prescription drugs release different neurotransmitters, scientists think that they all work on the brain in the same exact way: by releasing the "feel good" neurotransmitter dopamine first (Bragdon and Gamon 2000, 30). Increased levels of dopamine cause the person to feel very good—much lighter and happier. An addicted brain eventually changes, or rewires, and wants only one thing: the drug.

There are many ways that scientists are tackling the problem of prescription drug addiction and addiction overall: (1) by creating new drugs that are less addictive but just as helpful for treating problems with pain, sleeping, and attention/focus; (2) by discovering the genes that put some people at a greater risk for becoming addicted to drugs in the first place; (3) by figuring out the long-term effects these drugs have on the brain, potentially reversing the damage that has already been done.

References

Bragdon, Allen D., and David Gamon. 2000. *"Alcoholism, Etc: Triggering Transmitters:" Brains That Work a Little Bit Differently.* South Yarmouth, MA: Allen D. Bragdon Publishers, pp. 21–33.

National Institute on Drug Abuse. 2014, November. "Prescription Drug Abuse: Research Report Series." http://www.drugabuse.gov/publications/research-reports/prescription-drugs/.

National Institute on Drug Abuse. 2015. "Mind Over Matter—Prescription Drug Abuse." http://teens.drugabuse .gov/educators/nida-teaching-guides/mind-over-matter/ prescription-drug-abuse.

Maia Pujara looks at how peoples' brains "light up" to things like food, money, and drugs. She received her Ph.D. in neuroscience at the University of Wisconsin-Madison and completed her postdoctoral studies as an IRTA postdoctoral trainee at the National Institutes of Health. She now teaches at Sarah Lawrence College.

The Second-Best Time

Thomm Quackenbush

I was the kid who always avoided drugs. I never drank or smoked. Even when I had all my wisdom teeth pulled, I refused to fill my prescription for Vicodin.

As I grew up into college, psychiatric drugs replaced the recreational ones among my friends, and I resented the interference. I thought that I would never know who friends truly were, only who some chemical made them.

I refused to consider that I might need medication. True, I would weep with little antecedent. Yes, I would become irritated and could not articulate why. Okay, I would hide in my apartment because I could not motivate myself to leave, canceling plans at the last minute. And sure, I would become so lost in my branching worries that my attention span was crippled. That happens to everyone, I thought.

None of these were persistent conditions, so why would I make a big deal over them? They were easy for me to forget until they happened again—and they always happened again. When depression and anxiety overwhelmed me, I took them as accurate reflections of my life rather than understanding that imbalanced neurochemicals caused them.

I had suffered no trauma or abuse. I had a happy childhood. It made no sense for me to have a mental illness, so how could I?

I was into my adulthood, a year married, before I changed my mind. My wife tried to speak to me about some commonplace relationship friction. I plummeted into a numb spiral from which I could not extricate myself for days. I understood then that my choices were to admit that I had a problem or watch my marriage and the life containing it erode.

I finally accepted that what I felt was not normal. It is not normal to have to leave dinner because you've amplified some accidental slight until it is all you can hear. It is not normal to obsess over hypotheticals, most of which could never happen. It is not normal to cease to enjoy your life when nothing had outwardly changed.

My initial meeting with a nurse practitioner took twenty minutes. She asked me a few things and, based on these, diagnosed me with a mood disorder and sent me home with a sample of a medication. I felt cheated that seeking help at long last involved twenty questions and a blister pack. But, as I had the pills, I didn't want them to go to waste. In the worst-case scenario, taking them would prove that it was never medication that I needed.

Within days of taking the first, my life blossomed. I was never better able to understand and articulate my needs and thought processes. A weight had been lifted from me that I had grown so used to that I didn't register it. I had no idea how tightly I had been closed off from life.

I am a born writer, so I was hesitant to try medication. The persistent concern among creative types is that therapy will kill what makes us inspired. We are more than our neuroses. After starting treatment, I became more prolific and in touch with my muse because I was not clouded by disordered thinking. I could focus more fully on my work.

The first medication was not a success. It would have been close to a miracle if it had been. It was a marked improvement, but it also once resulted in nearly passing out after taking it at dinner and then sleeping for thirteen hours. I also gained weight that no amount of exercise could touch, but that was a secondary concern. Better to carry a few extra pounds than a ton of existential dread.

When I saw my nurse practitioner again, she switched my prescription. The new one did not cause me to fall asleep, and the extra weight vanished. However, in titrating to the prescribed dose, everything became so vivid that I broke down sobbing when the music on while I washed dishes moved me too deeply.

We halved my dosage, and I found, at last, my happy medium.

The medication didn't change who I was. It assisted me in remembering who I was supposed to be. It also did not cure me of my mental health issues. That isn't its purpose. It allowed me to be functional enough to gain healthier coping skills.

Months after starting on medication, I sought cognitive behavioral therapy, something I wouldn't have been able to do without. A year later, my therapist agreed that I had learned enough to no longer need to see her.

Bodies are not made perfect. I would not be ashamed to be diabetic or have an autoimmune disorder that required daily medication. Mental illness should be no different simply because it concerns one's brain and not one's pancreas.

I do not know if there will be a time in my life when I am going to no longer be on medication. As its effects have been entirely positive at the lower dosage—no side effects that would scare me away—I am inclined to stay with what works.

I reflected on situations in my life that would have gone otherwise if I had not allowed this help. I stayed in bad relationships and with the wrong jobs. I missed wonderful moments because my anxiety overruled my sense of adventure. I whiffed a dozen job interviews because I was too neurotic to perform. I mourn the life I could have had if I had accepted help, but I also have the skills now so I do not let this regret affect my future.

I wish I had tried medication earlier in my life, but at least I didn't wait a day more. As the saying goes, the best time to plant a tree is ten years ago. The second-best time is today.

Thomm Quackenbush is an author and educator in the Hudson Valley of New York, where he works with adjudicated youth. He writes the Night's Dream *series. His work is available at http:// thommquackenbush.com.*

Sick Full Time

Marissa Quenqua

"So, this means you have to pay out of pocket for everything?" my headache neurologist asks, sitting behind her solid oak desk in her private office near Columbus Circle. I am a patient at the Headache Institute in New York City, one of the only practices of its kind on the east coast.

"I'll just tell the office I saw you for fifteen minutes," she says, scribbling feverishly on her prescription pad. She hands me a stack of prescription refills. "I think we might be able to go longer than a month before your next visit!"

The receptionist at the front desk tells me that a fifteen-minute visit without health insurance costs $520. With coverage, I paid $40. I hand her my credit card and don't think about it too hard. I need to see this doctor. She makes another appointment in two months. I'm headed to the pharmacy next.

I've just lost my first full-time job as a production assistant at Penguin Random House. My health coverage ended along with it. I was diagnosed with chronic tension type and chronic vestibular migraine in July 2009, at twenty-four years old.

My chronic migraines showed up one day in May of that same year as a constant dizziness and pressure sensation in my skull. It was unlike anything I'd ever experienced. I woke up with it every morning, and it lasted all day. It was as if there was a screwdriver stuck in the back of my skull, radiating pressure to the front of it, or like there were a pile of bricks sitting on top of my head. I was used to dealing with a migraine or two per month since childhood, which felt more like being stabbed in the eye; sometimes, I'd vomit and I'd be out of commission for an afternoon. This was different: the symptoms never went away.

That spring I spent my weekends in the emergency room at Lenox Hill hospital, having CT scans and MRIs and blood work. I was told that everything had come back normal without the slightest variation and was sent home with a diagnosis of "headache." I felt insane. Walking home, the sidewalk looked like it was jumping up to meet me. I couldn't type on a computer for more than a few minutes without extreme dizziness. I went to an internist for an allergy panel, I went to an eye doctor, I went to an epilepsy specialist. They all found nothing. One neurologist suggested that the strange pressure and dizziness might be a migraine variant and wrote me a prescription for an antiseizure medication, which can sometimes work as a preventive: not in my case. That medication only made me dizzier.

I had to wait two months for an appointment at the Headache Institute, with constant symptoms the entire time. I took five baths a day because it was the only time I felt remotely comfortable. OTC pain meds did nothing for the dizziness or pressure. I had to keep reminding myself that all my scans and blood work were normal because I was convinced I had a brain tumor. I thought something that impacted my daily life so severely could not be benign. An internist gave me Xanax when he could find nothing else wrong with me. When I took that, I was still dizzy and had constant pressure in my skull. I just cared less about it.

On the morning of my appointment with the Headache Institute, I rode in a cab with my head on my girlfriend's lap because I was too dizzy to sit up straight. The buildings we drove by looked like they were warped; I was nauseous and felt like I was on hallucinogens. I'd used almost all of my vacation and personal time for the year trying to figure out what was wrong with me and was grateful to be approved for a twelve-week medical leave from work.

The neurologist at the Headache Institute gave me a formal diagnosis. The pressure sensation was a form of chronic tension-type migraine, and the dizziness was a form of chronic migraine called *vestibular migraine*. My migraines were "intractable," which is what they call them when they're constant. She reviewed my tests from the emergency room and said I had nothing more pressing wrong with me. I cried in her office because I knew it wasn't all in my mind. She wrote me a prescription for an antidepressant, which is used off label as a migraine preventive. It would take weeks to kick in, if it worked at all. There was no magic bullet. Treatment for my condition is trial and error.

After my medical leave elapsed, I was not cured. My doctor and I worked together, sometimes every week on the phone, to find a cocktail of meds that worked best. The treatments helped, but I still had constant symptoms. I was told I couldn't do my job part time, which is what my doctor recommended, so I returned to work full time in August. The screen time and stress and fluorescent lights only exacerbated my constant symptoms. I popped five muscle relaxers a day just to get through it and often had a painful, vomiting migraine every night. My neuro added a blood pressure medication, which can also work for migraine. It helped, but nothing brought me down to zero.

By the fall, it was clear I could no longer work full time. With the medications, I could walk down the street without dizziness or comfortably run errands but an eight-hour workday was too much. I was let go in November 2009, and my health insurance ended along with it. My income was from unemployment benefits alone. I am a first-generation college graduate who attended Sarah Lawrence College on a scholarship. I had no financial safety net.

"This is highway robbery," my pharmacist tells me.

My blood pressure medication now costs $75 a week. That's $300 a month for one prescription. I get $320 a week on unemployment. All of my medications together, which keep me functional if still unable to work, cost $450 a month. My parents assist me financially where they can, but they can't support me indefinitely. I run up thousands of dollars of credit card debt, something I vowed never to do. I moved to a lower-income neighborhood in Brooklyn with five roommates, and the pharmacist there chose to charge me less for my medication. I was surviving, but barely. I began temping, but the work was sporadic. I tried working as a hostess in a restaurant, but I wasn't making enough. I ended up back on the food stamp line I grew up on. When my unemployment benefits ended, I was evicted from my apartment. I got married in 2013 to a woman who works full time and that is the only reason I have health insurance to this day.

Eleven years later, I am still unable to work full time, although I've tried again several times over the years out of hope or financial necessity. After a few months, I always relapse and spend my workdays warding off dizziness and pain, my nights vomiting. In 2017, the last time I tried to work full time, my vision spliced completely in half during a work meeting: a zigzag of light appeared horizontally across my field of vision. It lasted for twenty minutes. I acted normal in front of my coworkers until I could hide in the bathroom until it passed. It's followed by a period of confusion—ocular migraine. It happened three times that week.

The most effective treatment for my chronic migraines aside from avoiding triggers and a consistent yoga practice is Botox injections. They're administered by a neurologist, approximately thirty-five shots to the face and head every three months. I was approved because I have fifteen or more migraine days per month and still have some level of constant symptoms. With my current insurance, I pay $0 out of pocket. Without insurance, it would cost me three grand.

What happened to me isn't something that should happen in the United States of America. As a kid born into a lower-income family, I followed the advice of every teacher I had.

I was passionate, studious, and dedicated. I received a scholarship to attend the college of my dreams. I moved to New York City and landed a full-time job with benefits at one of the most well-known publishing companies in the world. Then, at twenty-four, barely at the beginning of my career, I was sidelined by a health condition. Because we do not have universal health care, and my benefits were tied to my job, my foundation crumbled. I went from the brink of success to barely surviving within six months. Marriage shouldn't have been integral to a stable life, but that's exactly what happened.

Marissa Quenqua is a freelance writer on the brink of owning her first home, in Philadelphia, with her wife.

The Drug Supply Chain and the United States

Bob Roehr

Drop a cell phone and if the case splits open, it's easy to see the hundreds of silicone, metal, and plastic parts it's made of and believe that they came through a complex supply chain.

Cut open most pills and you are likely to see the same bland white interior. But if you look deeper, at the molecular and atomic levels, the structures vary greatly between an antibiotic that cures an infection, an antihypertensive that keeps blood pressure in check, and every other class of drug.

The active ingredient in each is the result of dozens of chemical processes, often under high temperature and pressure, that shape and reshape the atomic combinations toward that final drug product. The active ingredient is then combined with fillers, stabilizers, binders, coatings, and other materials that make sure it stays safe on the shelf, dissolves in the stomach or survives those acids to make it into the gut, and is absorbed by the body.

That production supply chain for these many raw materials and processes spreads across the world, and the distribution of those manufactured products is just as extensive. The

COVID-19 crisis has demonstrated just how interdependent we are for our health care products.

Most pharmaceutical companies are dedicated to making their drugs to the highest standards; a few are not so strict and are driven more by the bottom line.

The U.S. Food and Drug Administration (FDA) protects the integrity of those supply chains. It conducts rigorous surprise inspections of facilities that manufacture drugs certified for sale in the United States and works closely with regulators in Europe and Japan. However, some foreign governments require six weeks advance notice of such inspections, which gives wayward companies time to clean up their act.

Generic drugs are 92 percent of the prescriptions written in the United States, and almost all are produced overseas, primarily in India and China, because they have cheaper skilled labor, laxer environmental laws for the often-toxic chemical processes used in drug making, and government subsidies. Most of those drugs are of high quality but not all.

Several years ago, the FDA investigated consumer complaints about drugs produced in China and found systemic data manipulation by one large company. It banned twenty-nine drugs the company made but then had to exempt fourteen drugs because banning them would have resulted in a shortage in the United States, according to Rosemary Gibson in her 2018 book *Chinese Rx: Exposing the Risks of America's Dependence on China for Medicine* (Gibson 2018).

Unfortunately the consumer has little information in shopping for pharmaceuticals. Even the cheapest T-shirt has a label saying where it was made, but it is nearly impossible for you to find out where a drug was made.

Valisure is "an online pharmacy attached to an analytical laboratory" that tests every batch of a drug before distributing it to clients. "Currently we reject over 10 percent of on-market medication batches," its president David Light told a U.S. Senate hearing in June 2020 (Team Valisure 2020). The company was established in 2015 at the Yale Science Park and uses FDA standards for correct dosage, major active ingredients, proper dissolution, and the presence of carcinogens.

The company recently tested thirty-eight batches of the diabetes drug metformin from twenty-two different companies. Light said, "Our results showed that 42% of the batches analyzed (16 of 38) contained NDMA [which causes cancer in lab animals] exceeding the FDA's daily acceptable intake limit, with the highest detected amount over 16 times the permissible limit" (McMeekin, Abdoo, and Throckmorton 2020).

Civica Rx is a relatively new nonprofit company that was formed to address issues of drug shortages and quality. Its members include the Bill and Melinda Gates Foundation and health care systems, with about half the hospital beds in the United States.

"We made two really important decisions that worked out very well during the COVID-19 crisis. One was, we were never going to source our pharmaceutical ingredients from China, and the other was we were going to carry six months of safety stock for all of the drugs that we carry for our membership group," said Civica board chair Dan Liljenquist (Roehr 2020).

There is a bipartisan recognition that U.S. health care has become overly dependent on a supply chain that runs through China and an agreement that production of key drugs should be brought back to the United States. BARDA—the Biomedical Advanced Research and Development Agency—which is part of the U.S. Department of Health and Human Services (HHS), is perhaps the biggest and least known player.

Over the past year, BARDA has committed more than $10 billion for COVID-19 vaccine development. Their contracts generally carry a provision that some or all of a final product be manufactured in and initially distributed in the United States. In addition, more than a billion dollars has gone to create new production facilities for antibiotics, pain medicines, and other classes of drugs deemed crucial.

Ronald Piervincenzi, CEO of United States Pharmacopeia, a nonprofit that sets manufacturing quality standards used worldwide, is optimistic that the United States can become more competitive in its major problem area—generic drugs— by embracing continuous flow production techniques such as those envisioned for Phlow, Inc., one of the projects funded by BARDA.

He says groups like Civica, which are willing to make long-term agreements of five years or more to purchase set amounts of drugs at a set price, can increase the willingness of manufacturers to make investments in creating drug manufacturing capacity in the United States. Tax and investment incentives by government are another tool to support drug production.

Pharmaceutical industry veteran B. Frank Gupton, now head of Medicines for All, a nonprofit research group at Virginia Commonwealth University, says it took twenty to thirty years for the United States to lose much of its drug-manufacturing capacity to other countries: "It is going to take a while for us to bring it back. The question is, do we have the staying power to do that?"

References

Gibson, Rosemary. 2018. *Chinese Rx: Exposing the Risks of America's Dependence on China for Medicine.* New York: Prometheus Books.

McMeekin, Judith A., Mark Abdoo, and Douglas Throckmorton. 2020. "COVID-19 and Beyond: Oversight of the FDA's Foreign Drug Manufacturing Inspection Process." U.S. Food and Drug Administration. https:// www.fda.gov/news-events/congressional-testimony/ covid-19-and-beyond-oversight-fdas-foreign-drug-manufacturing-inspection-process-06022020.

Roehr, Bob. 2020. "Bringing Drug Production Home: How the US Is Rebuilding the Drug Supply Chain after Covid-19." September 21. *BMJ* 370: m3393. https:// doi.org/10.1136/bmj.m3393.

Team Valisure. 2020. "Valisure CEO Testimony at Senate
  Finance Committee on the FDA's Foreign Drug
  Manufacturing Inspection Process." *Valisure.* https://www
  .valisure.com/blog/valisure-news/valisure-ceo-testimony-at-
  senate-finance-committee-on-the-fda/.

*Bob Roehr is an award-winning freelance biomedical journalist
based in Washington, D.C.*

Can Information Technology Help Curb Prescription Drug Abuse?

Jeremy Summers

Just a few decades ago, Americans dreamed of a future with scientific advancements that improved every facet of their daily lives—better living through science. Along with fantasies of flying cars, robotic maids, and powdered meals, many Americans believed that one day, science would progress to the point that all one would need to do to cure an illness or improve one's health is take a pill.

Trying to fulfill these fantasies, scientists used advances in chemistry and biomedical research to start producing these types of pills. For many, these pills were a godsend—people with attention deficit hyperactivity disorder, for example, could now receive the extra chemical boost they needed, as could people with anxiety, sleep disorders, and many other illnesses.

But perhaps the makers of these pills were too successful in their mission. As the popularity and prevalence of prescription drugs rose, people began wholeheartedly subscribing to this complicated future of medicine. Capitalizing on this trend, big pharmaceutical companies began coming out with pills for every type of disorder, no matter how small or what other methods existed for treating the disorder.

In recent years, prescription drugs have become so effective and widespread that nearly 70 percent of Americans are on at least one prescription drug and more than 50 percent take two or more ("Nearly 7 in 10 Americans Take Prescription Drugs" 2013). Technological innovation had not only ushered in a new era of medicine but also introduced a new kind of scourge on the American people.

A 2013 report from the Trust for America's Health found that approximately 6.1 million Americans abuse or misuse prescription drugs. Overdose deaths from prescription drugs have at least doubled in more than twenty-nine states, where they now exceed vehicle-related deaths. Rates have tripled in ten of these states and quadrupled in four of them. These increases mean that more Americans now overdose from prescription drugs than from heroin, methamphetamine, and cocaine combined ("What Is a Public Health Approach to Reducing Prescription Drug Abuse?" 2013). But if advances in technology helped create this problem, can technology also help to solve it?

The same previously cited study found that the most commonly misused prescription drugs are painkillers, including some of the most popular: OxyContin, Percocet, and Vicodin. According to the study, men between the ages of twenty-five and fifty-four are most likely to abuse these drugs, though rates of female abusers are rapidly accelerating ("What Is a Public Health Approach to Reducing Prescription Drug Abuse?" 2013, 7–8).

The statistics make it clear that this has moved beyond a law enforcement problem and has become a national health care crisis. Approximately 50 Americans die from prescription painkiller overdoses each day, leading to more than 16,000 deaths and nearly half a million emergency room visits per year. Additionally, more than 70,000 children go to the emergency room every year for "medication poisoning," or when a child takes medicine prescribed for an adult ("What Is a Public Health Approach to Reducing Prescription Drug Abuse?" 2013).

So what role can technology play in this solution?

Many experts agree that digitizing medical records and "e-prescription" tools can help curb prescription drug abuse. By utilizing electronic records, doctors can limit drug diversion and doctor shopping and crack down on physicians who overprescribe or recommend drugs for nonmedical purposes. Implementation of information technology can address this problem immediately. More specifically, they can address the failures of current systems.

Currently, forty-nine states in the country have monitoring programs for prescription drugs. The problem is that the strategies in place are often too broad in scope, are woefully underfunded, and can even work against other systems fighting the same problem. Much of this, unfortunately, is due to a long history of inefficient bureaucracy, long paper trails, and lack of interconnectivity between different offices.

Much as it has done in countless other fields, information technology can address these failures. Perhaps the biggest improvement that can be yielded from implementation of information technology is the integration and connectivity of different public health systems networks so that all health care providers have access to these records and programs.

Information technology is not only the perfect tool to make these improvements and address perhaps the most serious health issue of the United States but also one that will help improve its economy.

This crisis extends beyond just health care. A study estimated that nearly every year, nonmedical use of prescription painkillers costs the U.S. economy roughly $53.4 billion—$42 billion lost in productivity, $8.2 billion in increased court costs, $2.2 billion for publicly funded drug abuse treatment programs, and $944 million in medical complications (Hansen et al. 2011).

Unfortunately, despite the fact that many of these systems are already in place to varying degrees, due to underfunding and lack of awareness, many states don't have access to them. For example, many state providers don't have access to prescription drug monitoring programs (PDMPs)—electronic databases that fight against doctor shopping, one of the most common methods people have for abusing prescription drugs. These programs track prescriptions by patients and automatically flag possible misuse by recognizing when multiple prescriptions of the same or similar drugs have been prescribed by different doctors for the same patient.

Additionally, many states have access to PDMPs but are not fully utilizing them. Many states also vary the requirements for reporting and determining who can access and report data. While all states except Missouri currently have PDMPs, only sixteen of those forty-nine require health care providers to use them ("Prescription Drug Abuse Now More Deadly than Heroin, Cocaine Combined" 2013).

Furthermore, only a mere 2 percent of health care providers nationwide have adopted PDMPs or other electronic monitoring systems. Pharmacies adopt these methods at a far higher rate, at nearly 78 percent, but the sad fact still remains in this day of technological innovation: only 2 percent of all controlled substances are prescribed electronically in the United States. These staggering numbers make it clearer than ever that most Americans are at risk for prescription drug abuse.

While it is clear that information technology can help curb prescription drug abuse, the biggest challenge to the implementation of these methods is not staunch opposition to them but rather a lack of organization or combined effort by the many different facets of the health care industry.

The real challenge in the coming years will be to involve prescribers, pharmacies, law enforcement agencies, insurance executives, and policy makers to work together to be part of the solution to this very real problem. Beyond expanding access to PDMPs, however, improved training for doctors and other health care providers is also key to curbing prescription drug abuse. Along these same lines, it is imperative that private and public insurance programs expand to cover a full range of substance abuse treatment programs to help cure patients of their addictions.

While there are still some very large hurdles to overcome in addressing this national health care crisis, society can take some comfort from the fact that information technology can clearly help curb prescription drug misuse and abuse. It seems, then, that it is just a matter of when—not if—we will utilize the benefits of technology to help us solve this problem.

References

Hansen, Ryan N., et al. 2011. "Economic Costs of Nonmedical Use of Prescription Opioids." *Clinical Journal of Pain.* 27(3): 194–202.

"Nearly 7 in 10 Americans Take Prescription Drugs." 2013. Mayo Clinic. http://newsnetwork.mayoclinic.org/ discussion/nearly-7-in-10-americans-take-prescription-drugs-mayo-clinic-olmsted-medical-center-find/.

"Prescription Drug Abuse Now More Deadly than Heroin, Cocaine Combined." 2013. *The Christian Science Monitor.* http://m.csmonitor.com/USA/Society/2013/1007/Prescription-drug-abuse-now-more-deadly-than-heroin-cocaine-combined.

"What Is a Public Health Approach to Reducing Prescription Drug Abuse." 2013. "Prescription Drug Abues: Strategies to Stop the Epidemic." *Trust for America's Health.* https://www2.deloitte.com/content/dam/Deloitte/us/Documents/life-sciences-health-care/us-lshc-Prescription-drug-abuse-102214.pdf.

Jeremy Summers is proposal manager at Moovit, in Clemmons, North Carolina. He has long been a freelance science writer whose work has appeared in Forbes, RealClearScience, *and* Truth About Trade, *among others. He is a graduate of Appalachian State University.*

HEART SAVER

Americ...
Ass...

Fighting...

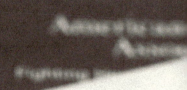

has part...
w... 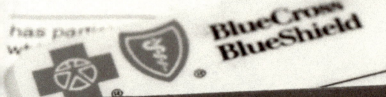 **BlueCross BlueShield** ®

KAISER PERMANENTE.

* Kaiser Foundation Health Plan, Inc.
Southern California Region

Prefix

00

Name:

UnitedHealthcar

Health Plan (808)... 911 ...

PacifiCare

The story of prescription drugs throughout history is, to a large extent, the story of individuals and organizations that have made significant contributions to the development and production of such products. This chapter provides an overview of some of the most important of those individuals and organizations.

Alliance for Safe Online Pharmacies

Opioid abusers and addicts have access to the drugs they want and need through a number of avenues. One such source of drugs is the Internet. According to some estimates, there may be anywhere between 35,000 and 50,000 online pharmacies worldwide willing to sell opioids and other drugs to individuals of any age. When the U.S. Department of Justice closed down just one site in 2017, it found that the company involved, AlphaBay, had a list of more than 200,000 customers and an inventory of more than 250,000 illegal and/or toxic drugs for sale. In response to this problem, the Alliance for Safe Online Pharmacies (ASOP) was established in 2009 to monitor websites that maintain such operations. ASOP estimates that 97 percent of active online sellers of drugs and medications do not comply with relevant national and international laws and regulations dealing with patient safety. Without guidance from some reliable source, such as the ASOP, the average consumer

A set of medical prescription cards. (David Tonelson/Dreamstime.com)

has virtually no way of knowing which Internet sites are legitimate sources of safe drugs and which are not.

The mission of ASOP, therefore, is to protect patient safety in the purchase of drugs online. The organization is an international association with headquarters in Washington, D.C. It is classified as a 501(c)(4) social welfare organization that is supported financially by contributions from companies, nonprofit organizations, and trade associations, along with voluntary donations and contributions from interested individuals.

ASOP has two categories of participants: members and observers. Membership, in turn, is divided into two classes: board members and general members. Board members establish policy and carry out the organization's day-to-day operations. General members advise the board and participate equally in all policy decisions. Those decisions are not voted upon but are made by consensus of all members participating in the discussion. Current members of the organization come from a variety of fields and include organizations such as the American Pharmacists Association, Amgen, Eli Lilly, European Alliance for Safe Access to Medicines, Generic Pharmaceutical Association, Italian Medicines Agency, Johnson & Johnson, Partnership for Drug-Free Kids, Takeda Pharmaceuticals, and U.S. Pharmacopeial Convention.

The observers group consists of organizations to whom ASOP turns for specialized advice on specific topics or that provide information to the organization on a volunteer basis. Observers do not vote on ASOP policies or practices. Some organizations currently serving as observers are the American Association of Colleges of Pharmacy, Federation of State Medical Boards, National Health Council, Partnership for Safe Medicines, and Rx-360.

ASOP's activities focus on the collection of information about the sale of medications on the Internet, information that is then used to educate health care providers, policy makers, drug manufacturers, and suppliers, and the general public. In collaboration with its members and observers, the organization develops policy solutions for issues related to online pharmaceutical marketing that it recommends to legislative and administrative agencies at all levels of government.

ASOP uses primarily two methods in its educational efforts: direct (usually video) presentations and electronic publications. Examples of the former are presentations made by ASOP staff at the Asia-Pacific Economic Cooperation Life Sciences Innovation Forum Workshop on Medical Products Safety and Public Awareness and Establishing of a Single Point of Contact System in Seoul, Korea; at the Partnership for Safe Medicines' Interchange 2011; and at the PDA/FDA Pharmaceutical Supply Chain Conference: Patients Impacted by Supply Chain Dangers.

Some of the many electronic publications on Internet pharmacies available on ASOP's website are "How to Protect Yourself and Your Loved Ones Online," "Infographic about the Origin of Counterfeit Drugs in G8 Member Countries," "LegitScript's Legitimate Online Pharmacy List," "Legitscript's Website URL Verification Tool," "Making the Internet Safe for Patients," "National Association of Boards of Pharmacy's VIPPS List," "Online Pharmacy 101: What You Need to Know," and the U.S. Food and Drug Administration's "Know Your Online Pharmacy" tool.

ASOP's website is also a valuable resource for reports, news items, and other documents about the availability of medications online. Some of these resources come from ASOP itself, others from government sources, others from academic sources, and still others from partner resources. The types of documents that one might find in this section of the website are articles such as "Vaccine Shortages and Suspect Online Pharmacy Sellers," "ASOP One-Pager on the Online Pharmacy Safety Act," "Consumer Fact Sheet: FDA Online Medicine Buying Guide," "The Japanese Rogue Internet Pharmacy Market," and "Assessing the Problem of Counterfeit Medications in the United Kingdom."

Bayer AG

Most historians acknowledge German pharmacist Friedrich Sertürner as the discoverer of morphine in 1803, one of the most important analgesics available to the medical profession. Similar accolades are offered for the work of Belgian chemist Paul Janssen for his 1960 discovery of an even more powerful pain reliever: fentanyl. And credit for the synthesis of yet another powerful analgesic, oxycodone, is given to German chemists Martin Freund and Jakob Edmund Speyer, in 1916. So who deserves credit for the discovery of so many of the best-selling, most widely used prescription drugs in the world, compounds such as rivaroxaban (Xarelto), drospirenone/ethinyl estradiol (e.g., Yasmin, YAZ), ciprofloxacin (Cipro), and aflibercept (Eylea)?

The simplest answer to that question is researchers at the Bayer Pharmaceuticals company in Germany. Today, and for some time in the recent past, drug discovery has no longer been the result of some individual researcher working in a lab. Instead, it occurs through the efforts of dozens or hundreds of researchers working at pharmaceutical companies of many sizes, who work for many years at the cost of hundreds of millions of dollars to find a new prescription drug. Among the largest of these drug companies today are Pfizer, Roche, Novartis, Merck, GlaxoSmithKline, and Johnson & Johnson. From a historical standpoint, however, no drug company is of as much significance as Bayer Pharmaceuticals.

The Bayer company was founded in 1863 in Barmen, Germany, by Friedrich Baeyer and his business partner, Johann Weskott. Baeyer was a chemical products salesman with a special interest in dyes, while Weskott was a master dyer. (Baeyer changed his name to its present spelling when he was still a young man.) The company, Bayer AG, was formed to make and sell dyes, with Weskott in charge of production and Bayer in charge of sales and marketing. Perhaps the most significant feature of the new company was its decision to focus on the manufacture of synthetic dyes rather than developing dyes from natural materials, as was largely the approach to dyes at the time. The critical breakthrough in this regard occurred in 1884, when the Bayer company decided to establish a research laboratory for the discovery of new chemical products. Although the invention, production, and sale of dyes was still the major focus of the Bayer business, experiments in other fields became more popular. The most important product resulting from this research was a commercial form of one of the oldest of all known analgesics: acetylsalicylic acid. By making modest changes to the chemical structure of this substance, Bayer researchers came up with a valuable new pain killer, which they patented in 1899 under the name *aspirin*.

With its new success in the field of drugs, Bayer turned more and more attention to the development—if not the actual discovery—of other commercial products. In 1898, it began production of a commercial form of heroin to be advertised and sold as an drug for the treatment of coughs and colds, pneumonia, tuberculosis, and a host of other common ailments. Five years later, in 1903, the company began producing another very successful drug, diethylbarbituric acid, sold under the trade name Veronal and recommended as a mild hypnotic for improved sleeping patterns. A modest chemical change in that compound then resulted in the production of another new drug, phenobarbital, which became popular for the treatment of epilepsy and other conditions.

In 1925, the Bayer company became involved in what is probably its darkest period in history. It joined with five other large chemical companies to form a new corporation, IG Farben, which shortly became the largest commercial enterprise in Germany. The company became an essential cog in the Nazi German war machine throughout the 1930s. Among many of the new companies' least admirable projects during the war were some important drug discoveries made at former Bayer facilities. One of these was prontosil (also, Prontosil), the first antibacterial drug to become commercially available (1932).

Another successful invention was an antimalarial drug known as chloroquine (later sold at Resochin). The company donated three million doses of the drug in 2020 for possible therapeutic uses against the novel coronavirus.

At the end of World War II, the Allied nations decided to disband IG Farben and break it into numerous small companies. When that plan turned out to be impractical for economic reasons, the decision was made to remake the company in the form of a dozen smaller corporations, one of which was Farbenfabriken Bayer AG. In 1972, the company changed its name again, this time to simply Bayer AG.

Leading into the twenty-first century, Bayer felt many of the pressures experienced by corporations worldwide: to grow and expand. It began to acquire existing companies involved with the wide variety of products already part of the Bayer agenda. Finally, in 2003, Bayer reimagined itself as a holding company, Bayer AG, with four major components: Bayer Pharmaceuticals, Bayer Consumer Health, Bayer Crop Science, and Animal Health. Among its leading pharmaceutical products in 2020 were Xarelto, Eylea, Adempas, Xofigo, Stivarga, Mirena-Produktfamilie, Kogenate/Kovaltry/Jivi, Nexavar, YAZ/Yasmin/Yasminelle, Glucobay, Adalat, Aspirin Cardio, Betaferon/Betaseron, Gadavist/Gadovist, and Stellant.

Drug Enforcement Administration

The U.S. Drug Enforcement Administration (DEA) has a long bureaucratic history. Its original predecessors were the Bureau of Narcotics, created within the Department of the Treasury in 1930, and the Bureau of Drug Abuse Control, established as part of the Food and Drug Administration in 1966. The two agencies were then combined in 1968 with the creation of the Bureau of Narcotics and Dangerous Drugs (BNDD) by Reorganization Plan No. 1 and placed within the Department of Justice. Five years later, another reorganization plan created the DEA in the merger of the BNDD with four other drug-related agencies: the Office of National Narcotics Intelligence in the Department of Justice; the drug investigation arm of the U.S. Customs Services, in the Department of the Treasury; the Narcotics Advance Research Management Team, in the Executive Office of the President; and the Office of Drug Abuse Law Enforcement, also in the Department of Justice. At the time it was created, DEA had 1,470 special agents and a budget of less than $75 million. In 2019, those numbers had risen to 10,169 employees, including over 4,600 special agents, over 600 diversion investigators, nearly 800 intelligence research specialists, and close to 300 chemists. Its FY 2019 budget was $3.136 billion and maintains 239 district offices in 23 divisions in the United States and 91 overseas offices in 68 countries.

The mission of the DEA is to enforce the controlled substance laws and regulations of the U.S. government and to bring to justice those individuals and organizations that violate those laws and regulations. In achieving this objective, the agency carries out a number of specific activities:

- investigating and preparing for prosecution violators of controlled substance laws operating at interstate and international levels
- investigating and preparing for prosecution individuals and gangs who use violence to terrorize individuals and communities in their sale and trafficking of drugs
- managing a national drug intelligence program, in cooperation with other federal agencies, as well as state, local, and international agencies, to collect, analyze, and distribute information on drug activities
- seizing assets that can be shown to be associated with illicit drug activities
- enforcing, in particular, the provisions of the Controlled Substances Act of 1970 and its later amendments pertaining to the manufacture and distribution of substances listed under that Act

- working with state and local agencies to deal with interstate and international illicit drug activities
- working with the United Nations, Interpol, and other organizations on matters related to international drug control programs

DEA activities are organized under two major categories: law enforcement and education and prevention. The major activities of law enforcement are the Diversion Control Division, El Paso Intelligence Center, Forensic Sciences, and Intelligence Program. Those of the education and prevention field are Community Outreach, the Red Ribbon Campaign, National Prescription Drug Takeback Day, and DEA 360 Strategy. Details of each of these programs are available on the DEA website, at dea.gov.

Another important way in which the DEA carries out its mandates is through task forces. A task force is a consortium of DEA and other federal officers, along with state and local law enforcement personnel designed to work on some specific drug enforcement issue. The earliest task forces, in the 1970s, were relatively informal groups operating without any official authorization or control. That approach changed in 1986, when the Anti-Drug Abuse Act provided official authorization for the organization of such groups. Today, more than 200 task forces exist in almost every state of the United States and Puerto Rico.

The DEA website provides a variety of useful data and documents dealing with drug enforcement issues in the United States. Three of the most important data sets include information on drug labs in the United States, domestic arrests, and meth lab incidents. Examples of the documents available on the DEA website are "The 2018 Heroin Signature Program," "Prescription Opioid Threat in Pennsylvania, 2020," "The Drug Situation in Delaware," "Fentanyl Flow to the United States," "Drug Caused Deaths in the LA Field Division," "Vaping and Marijuana Concentrates," and Fact Sheets on a host of drugs, including synthetic opioids, stimulants, salvia divinorum, psilocybin, oxycodone, and morphine. The website also contains a helpful collection of images relating to drug issues, such as images of several types of drugs, a collection of education and outreach videos, several press conferences on relevant topics, special DEA-related events, and important public service announcements about drug issues.

Carl Durham (1892–1974)

Durham was coauthor with Senator Hubert Humphrey (D-MN) of an amendment to the Federal Food, Drug, and Cosmetic Act of 1938 that required certain types of drugs to be sold only through prescription and to be labeled as noting that they were available only by prescription. The Act was significant because prior to its adoption, there was no legal or formal process for distinguishing between drugs that might pose a threat to one's health or life and those that were completely safe to take, the classes of drugs now known as prescription and over-the-counter drugs, respectively. In a sense, then, Durham and Humphrey may be called the *fathers of prescription drugs*. Additional provisions of the Durham-Humphrey amendment allowed a pharmacist to refill a prescription without receiving additional instructions from the prescriber and permitted prescriptions to be ordered verbally as well as in writing.

Carl Thomas Durham was born at White Cross, in Orange County, North Carolina, on August 28, 1892. He was the oldest of the six children of Claude and Delia Ann Durham (née Lloyd). Carl Durham attended the local elementary school in White Cross before continuing his education at the privately run Manndale Academy at Saxapahaw, just west of White Cross. In the summer of 1913, at the age of twenty-one, Durham began work as an apprentice pharmacist at Eubanks Drugstore in Chapel Hill. Three years later, he had achieved sufficient experience to qualify for the pharmacy program at the University of North Carolina, from which he graduated in 1917. He then enlisted in the U.S. Navy, following the United

States' entering World War I. Durham served as a pharmacist's mate for one year, before leaving the navy at the end of the war and returning to the Eubanks Drugstore as a professional pharmacist.

Even as a young man, Durham was active in civic and religious groups, serving as a deacon in his church and as president of his Bible class at the church. His first foray into politics occurred in 1921, when he was elected to the Chapel Hill Board of Alderman, a post he held until 1930. He was also elected to the Chapel Hill School Board, where he served from 1924 to 1938, and the Orange County Board of Commissioners, where he was a member from 1932 to 1938. Throughout this period, Durham continued to work as a pharmacist at Eubanks.

In 1938, Representative William B. Umstead, from North Carolina's Sixth Congressional District, retired and the candidate selected by the Democratic Party to replace him died before the election was held. With less than two weeks before the election, the party then selected Durham to run for the post, and he was elected without Republican opposition. Durham later ran and was reelected ten more times before finally retiring from the body in 1961. While serving in the House, his major position was chair of the Joint Committee on Atomic Energy in the 82nd and 85th Congresses. He also served on the House Military Affairs and Armed Services Committees. During his tenure, he was acknowledged by the Library of Congress as "the only pharmacist in Congress," although that accolade was not precisely true since his cosponsor for the prescription drug bill, Senator Hubert Humphrey, also had earned his license in pharmacy.

During the latter portion of his career, he became especially interested and active in issues related to the use of atomic energy, which had arisen at the end of World War II with the debate over control of the powerful new source of energy. Durham was a persistent spokesperson for the position that control of the new energy source should remain in civilian hands, in contrast to the position of military leaders, who hoped to maintain control over atomic power themselves. Durham was a delegate to the Atoms for Peace Conference held in Geneva in 1955 and attended the initial meeting of the Atomic Energy Agency in Vienna two years later.

After he retired from Congress in 1961, Durham was named honorary president of the American Pharmaceutical Association and hired as a special consultant to the organization. An article in the association's publication, *Drug Topics*, observed that if an award existed for the pharmacist who had performed the greatest service for his country, it would have to go to Carl Durham. Durham died in Durham, North Carolina, on April 29, 1974, and was interred at the Antioch Baptist Church Cemetery, in Chapel Hill. He had been married twice and had eight children and twenty-six grandchildren.

Hubert Humphrey (1911–1978)

Humphrey was one of the leading members of the Democratic Party during the 1960s and 1970s. He served as vice president under President Lyndon B. Johnson from 1965 to 1969, was twice U.S. senator from the state of Minnesota (1949–1964 and 1971–1978), and was the nominee of the Democratic Party for president of the United States in 1968, when he lost to Richard M. Nixon. One of his many legislative accomplishments while serving in the Senate was the cosponsorship of the Durham-Humphrey Amendment to the Federal Food, Drug, and Cosmetic Act of 1938 with Representative Carl Durham, of North Carolina. That Act was of considerable importance because, for the first time in U.S. history, a category of drugs was created whose use was deemed to involve sufficient risk to require that they not be freely available over the counter in a pharmacy. Such drugs, according to the Act, could be dispensed only by prescription that could be filled at a registered pharmacy. The Act, therefore, made a clear distinction between prescription drugs and other types of medications that could be sold without a prescription, the so-called over-the-counter drugs.

Hubert Horatio Humphrey Jr. was born in the tiny town of Wallace, South Dakota, on May 27, 1911. His parents were Ragnild Kirstine (née Sannes), a Norwegian immigrant, and Hubert Horatio Humphrey Sr. ("H.H."), a pharmacist. When Hubert Jr. was still young, his family moved to the slightly larger town of Doland, South Carolina, where his father opened a drug store. The business struggled there, and H.H. tried his best to keep it going by selling anything he could think of, from paint to rakes to toys to chocolates. By the beginning of the Great Depression, however, Humphrey's Drug Store had been forced into foreclosure, and H.H. was forced to sell the business and try his luck elsewhere, this time in the still slightly larger town of Huron, South Dakota. He had greater success there, and the business continues to operate today under the management of another family member, drawing its business more as a tourist site than as a purveyor of medicine. It was behind the soda fountain at the drug store that the young Humphrey had his introduction to the field of pharmacy during his after-school hours.

After completing high school in Doland, Humphrey enrolled at the University of Minnesota, with hopes of earning his doctorate in political science and becoming a college professor. With the difficult financial times developing, he had to leave Minnesota after the first year and continued his studies instead at the Capitol College of Pharmacy, in Denver, from which he earned his two-year licensure program in six months. He then returned to Huron to help his father in the drug store, realizing that pharmacy might be the career in which he would remain.

By 1937, however, the nation's economic situation had begun to improve, and Humphrey was convinced that he could not spend the rest of his life in the Huron drug store. So he returned to Minnesota, where he earned his bachelor's degree in political science, in 1939. He then moved on to Louisiana State University, from which he received his master's degree a year later. In 1940, he left Louisiana to return to Minnesota, where he enrolled as a doctoral student in political science. He never went very far in that program, however, as circumstances conspired to interrupt his long-held dream of earning a doctorate. The first of those circumstances was the outbreak of World War II, prompting Humphrey to attempt enlisting, first in the U.S. Navy and then in the U.S. Army. He was rejected multiple times by both arms of the service for a variety of physical problems, and he decided, instead, to involve himself in a variety of war-related activities, such as work on the War Manpower Commission.

In 1943, while serving as a professor of political science at Macalester College, in St. Paul, Humphrey decided to run for mayor of Minneapolis. He lost the election by a narrow margin but achieved greater success two years later, when he was elected with 61 percent of the vote. He served in that office until 1948, the year in which he made one of the most famous speeches at a Democratic National Convention in modern history. In that speech, he made an unabashed plea for greater progress in the field of civil rights, an issue that was, at the time, tearing the Democratic Party apart. The speech placed Humphrey on the national state in Democratic politics, a place where he remained for the rest of his life.

Humphrey followed up his success at the Democratic convention by gaining election to the U.S. Senate from the state of Minnesota in the fall of 1948, defeating incumbent Republican senator Joseph H. Ball with 60 percent of the vote. He was reelected twice more, in 1954 and 1960.

Throughout much of the last half of his tenure in the Senate, Humphrey was also angling for higher office, either that of the presidency or that of the vice presidency. He never achieved these goals by way of an election, but he did become vice president on January 20, 1965, when he was chosen by President Lyndon B. Johnson to fill that office, which had been vacant since the assassination of President John F. Kennedy fourteen months earlier. When Johnson decided not to run for another term in 1968, Humphrey at last had his chance for the highest office in the land, when he was chosen as the Democratic nominee for the presidency at the 1968 national convention. In the general election, Humphrey garnered 42.7 percent of the popular vote compared to 43.4 percent for Republican nominee Richard M. Nixon. But that small difference translated into a landslide for Nixon, who earned 301 electoral votes compared to 191 for Humphrey. (Alabama governor George Wallace won 46 electoral votes in the Deep South).

After the 1968 election, Humphrey returned to teaching at Macalester and the University of Minnesota. Then, in something of a twist of fate, he decided to run once more for the U.S. Senate from the state in the election of 1970, a contest he won handily. He was reelected in 1976 but was unable to serve out his term. In 1977, he announced that he had terminal bladder cancer, a disease from which he died on January 13, 1978, at his home in Waverly, Minnesota. Although the flashpoint of considerable political controversy throughout his career, Humphrey was generally well liked and widely admired as a politician who always fought fervently for the causes in which he believed, the happy warrior of modern American politics, as his Senate colleagues were wont to call him.

Paul Janssen (1926–2003)

In a biographical sketch about Janssen's life on the *Scientific American* blog, Janssen is described as "the most prolific drug inventor of all time." He and the research teams that worked at his company, Janssen Pharmaceutica, have been credited with the synthesis of at least eighty new drugs. At the time of his death in 2003, Janssen himself held more than one hundred patents on new bioactive compounds. Among the most important of his many discoveries was the opioid fentanyl, sold under a number of brand names, best known of which is Sublimaze. Sublimaze is most widely used as an anesthetic for surgical and other medical procedures. In the early 2000s, fentanyl became very popular among drug abusers and addicts. It gained this popularity because it is much more potent than many other opioids, about one hundred times more potent than an equal quantity of morphine, for example. It also tends to act more quickly than other popular opioids. In some cases, fentanyl is also easier to obtain on the streets than are heroin, morphine, or other opioids. In the United States, fentanyl is classified as a Schedule II drug, a drug with a high potential for abuse, potentially leading to severe psychological or physical dependence.

Paul Adriaan Jan Janssen was born on September 12, 1926, in Turnhout, Belgium. His father was Jan Constant Janssen, a physician, and his mother Margriet Fleerackers Janssen. Biographers note that Janssen's later career as a drug innovator was strongly influenced by two events early in his life. First, his father, already interested in developing his own business, obtained the rights to the sale of Hungarian-produced drugs in the Belgian Congo. That experience is thought to have made Paul Janssen aware of the possible economic benefits of drug research. The second event was the death of his younger sister of tubercular meningitis when she was only four years of age. That event appears to have convinced Janssen that he should devote his life to the discovery of substances that could be used in the treatment of disease.

Janssen attended secondary school at the Jesuit-run St Jozef College in Turnhout, where he decided to pursue a medical career. On graduation, he matriculated at the Faculté Universitaire Notre Dame de la Paix in Namur, no small accomplishment in and of itself given the wartime conditions then existing in Western Europe. At Notre Dame, he continued his premedical curriculum, concentrating in chemistry, biology, and physics. After receiving his B.S. in natural sciences in 1945, Janssen continued his studies at the Catholic University of Louvain, from where he earned his M.D. in 1951. His studies there were interrupted briefly when he traveled to the United States for six months to visit a number of pharmaceutical companies.

Over the next two years, Janssen served his required term of service in the Belgian army while simultaneously working in the Institute of Pharmacology at the University of Cologne, in Germany. In 1953, Janssen decided that it was time to strike out on his own and found a pharmaceutical research company. He and his first four employees established a laboratory on the third floor of his father's business in Turnhout and began a remarkable career of drug creation. Within the first year of operation, the Janssen team had synthesized about 500 new compounds and, two years later, more than 1,100 new substances. Obviously, not every new discovery turned out to have a medical application (the vast majority of them did not). But one of his earliest discoveries, ambucetamide, was found to have significant antispasmodic effects and was put to use for the treatment of menstrual pain. The new drug established Janssen's company as a serious organization to be reckoned with in the drug market. Some of the other drugs discovered during the company's early years were isopropamide, used for the treatment of peptic ulcers and gastrointestinal pain; diphenoxylate, used in the treatment of diarrhea; and the painkiller dextromoramide.

In 1957, Janssen's company, now called N.V. Research Laboratorium Dr. C. Janssen, had outgrown its Turnhout location and had moved to a former military camp at Beerse, less than five miles from Turnhout. There, research continued at an impressive rate, with the discovery of more than a dozen important drugs over the next five years. In 1961, Janssen agreed to sell his company to the giant pharmaceutical firm Johnson & Johnson, with the understanding that Janssen's own laboratory would be allowed to continue its own line of research independent from the parent company's control. The list of drugs eventually discovered by the Janssen research team includes important compounds such as disopromine, cinnarizine, moperone, trifluperidol, pipamperone, benperidol, dehydrobenzperiodol, spiperone, fluspirilene, pimozide, bromperidol, penfluridol, bromperidol decanoate, risperodone, haloperidol, levamisole, miconazole, and mebendazole. The last

four of these compounds are currently included on the World
Health Organization's List of Essential Medicines. Janssen died
in Rome, Italy, on November 11, 2003, while attending the
celebration of the 400th anniversary of the founding of the
Pontifical Academy of Sciences, of which he had been a member since 1990. His work has been recognized by a number of
honors and awards, including the Canada Gairdner Award, one
of the highest honors given to researchers in the field of medicine and health. In 2005, he was chosen the second "greatest
Belgian" of all time (after Father Damien) in a poll conducted
by Belgian public TV broadcaster Canvas, public radio broadcaster Radio 1, and newspaper *De Standaard*.

Kaiser Family Foundation

The Kaiser Family Foundation (KFF) was established 1948
with a grant from American industrialist and father of modern
shipbuilding technology, Henry J. Kaiser. The Foundation has
a long and complex history that has gone through a number of
transitions since Kaiser's death in 1967. Today, the organization prefers to call itself KFF because it is no longer a foundation nor associated with the major health care function of a
similar name, Kaiser Permanente. Since its most recent trans-
formation, its goal has been "to build an institution that plays
a special role as a trusted source of information in a health care
world dominated by vested interests" (https://www.kff.org/
history-and-mission).

KFF's current activities fall into four major categories: policy
analysis, polling, journalism, and communication. Some specific initiatives in each area are The Program on Medicaid and
the Uninsured, The Program on the Health Care Marketplace,
The Program on Medicare Policy, The Program on the ACA
(Affordable Care Act), The Racial Equity and Health Policy
Program, Women's Health Policy, State Health Reform and
Data, and The Global Health & HIV Policy Program (policy
analysis); The Public Opinion & Survey Research Program

(polling); Kaiser Health News and the Kaiser Media Fellow-ships in Health Reporting (journalism); and Social Impact Media (communication).

Research and reporting from KFF fall into about eleven major areas: COVID-19, disparities policy, global health policy, health costs, health reform, HIV/AIDS, Medicaid, Medicare, private insurance, uninsured, and women's health policy. Some of the most useful pieces of information provided by KFF come in the form of tables, graphs, charts, interactives, slides, and other creative forms of media. For example, the interactive chart on state health facts provides information for every state in the United States on a range of topics, including demographics and the economy, disparities, healthy costs and budgets, health coverage and uninsured, health insurance and managed care, health reform, health status, HIV/AIDS, Medicaid and Children's Health Insurance Program, Medicare, providers and service use, and women's health. This chart can be found at https://www.kff.org/statedata/.

Some of the many of KFF's reports on prescription drug issues are "What's the Latest on Prescription Drug Proposals from the Trump Administration, Congress, and the Biden Campaign?," "Prescription Drugs" (2020), "Most People Are Unlikely to See Drug Cost Savings from President Trump's 'Most Favored Nation' Proposal," "10 FAQs on Prescription Drug Importation," "Public Opinion on Prescription Drugs and Their Prices," "Pricing and Payment for Medicaid Prescription Drugs," "JAMA Forum: Trump vs Biden on Health Care," "States Are Shifting How They Cover Prescription Drugs in Response to COVID-19," and "Understanding the Medicaid Prescription Drug Rebate Program."

William Proctor Jr. (1817–1874)

Proctor is widely regarded as the father of pharmacy. According to one biographer, he "made no fortune, started no great pharmaceutical firm, discovered no new wonder drug, founded no school or journal. Yet, upon his death in 1874, he was hailed as the father of American pharmacy, a title never challenged since" (https://www.jstor.org/stable/41111692).

William Proctor Jr. was born on May 3, 1817, in Baltimore, Maryland. He was the youngest of nine children of Isaac and Rebecca Proctor (née Farquhar). Isaac was engaged in the mercantile trade in Baltimore, dying of yellow fever when William was three years of age. The boy was then placed in a school run by the Friends, of whom the Proctors had long been adherents. At the age of fourteen, William was offered a position as an apprentice to one Henry M. Zollickoffer in a pharmacy shop in Philadelphia, which he accepted. At the time, pharmacy was a somewhat disorganized business that relied on the preparation and distribution of compounds in the traditional materia medica. Proctor's willingness and ability to learn about the occupation soon caught the attention of older members of the field, and he was offered increasingly responsible positions in the field. He was invited to enroll in the Philadelphia College of Pharmacy, from which he graduated in 1837. Seven years later, he opened his own shop in Philadelphia, where, according to his biographer, he "struggled . . . for the rest of his life as a pharmacist" (https://www.jstor.org/stable/41111692).

Proctor's shop was somewhat different from most existing facilities of its type at the time. In addition to providing drugs to his customers, he devoted substantial amounts of time to original research in a laboratory at the rear of the shop. He regularly reported the results of his studies in papers published in the young *Journal of the Philadelphia College of Pharmacy* (later to become the *American Journal of Pharmacy*). The results of Proctor's research were also instrumental in updating the 1820 version of the U.S. Phamacopoeia, the standard collection of drug formulations in the country.

Proctor found greater success within the growing profession of pharmacy then in his commercial efforts. At the age of twenty-nine, in 1846, he was appointed the first permanent professor of pharmacy in the United States at the Philadelphia

College of Pharmacy. Two years later, he also joined the staff of the *American Journal of Pharmacy* as its assistant editor. In 1850, he was promoted to editor of the journal. During the same period, in 1849, Proctor published the first textbook on pharmacy produced in the United States (*Lectures on Practical Pharmacy*, London: J. and A. Churchill, 1883).

Proctor's own experiences in the profession of pharmacology convinced him of the need for more formal training for practitioners in the field. In the late 1840s, he wrote extensively in support of the creation of a professional association of pharmacists, a hope that was realized in 1851 with the founding of the American Pharmaceutical Association, an organization that continues today under the title of the American Pharmacists Association.

As his health began to fail in the late 1860s, he began to abandon some of his professional responsibilities. He resigned his position as professor of pharmacy in 1866 and handed over his job as editor of the journal in 1871. He planned, at that point, to devote his time to his own business, but events did not turn out in quite that way. When his good friend and fellow teacher Edward Parrish died in 1872, Proctor decided to return to his post at the Philadelphia College of Pharmacy, where he continued until shortly before his death. He died in Philadelphia on February 10, 1874. Proctor was later honored by the American Pharmacists Association on a number of occasions, most notably the erection of a statue in his honor in the foyer of the Washington headquarters of the American Pharmacists Association.

Friedrich Sertürner (1783–1841)

While still a young pharmacist's apprentice, Sertürner isolated the psychoactive agent morphine from the opium plant. His accomplishment is especially important, because it was not only the first such agent extracted from opium but also the first alkaloid obtained from any plant. Sertürner named his new discovery after the Greek god of dreams, Morpheus, for its powerful analgesic and sedative properties.

Friedrich Wilhelm Adam Ferdinand Sertürner was born in Neuhaus, Prussia, on June 19, 1783. His parents were in service to Prince Friedrich Wilhelm, who was also his godfather. When both his father and the prince died in 1794, he was left without means of support and, therefore, was apprenticed to a court apothecary by the name of Cramer. One of the topics in which he became interested in his new job was the chemical composition of opium, a plant that had long been known for its powerful analgesic and sedative properties. By 1803, he had extracted from opium seeds a white crystalline powder clearly responsible for the pharmacological properties of the plant. He named the new substance morphine and proceeded to test its properties, first on stray animals available at the castle and later on his friends and himself. His friends soon withdrew from the experiments because, while pleasurable enough in its initial moderate doses, the compound ultimately caused unpleasant physical effects, including nausea and vomiting. Sertürner continued, however, to test the drug on himself, unaware of its ultimate addictive properties.

Sertürner was awarded his apothecary license in 1806 and established his own pharmacy in the Prussian town of Einbeck. In addition to operating his business, he continued to study the chemical and pharmacological properties of morphine for a number of years. His work drew little attention from professional scientists, however, and he eventually turned his attention to other topics, including the development of improved firearms and ammunition. During the last few years of his life, he became increasingly depressed about his failure to invoke the interest of the scientific community in his research on opium. He withdrew into his own world and turned to morphine for comfort against his disillusionment with what he saw as the failure of his life. He did receive some comfort in 1831, when he was awarded a Montyon Prize by the Académie Française, sometimes described as the forerunner of the Nobel Prizes, with its cash award of 2,000 francs. By the time of his death in Hamelin, Prussia, on February 20, 1841, however, the scientific world in general had still not appreciated the enormous significance of his research on morphine.

Alexander "Sasha" Shulgin (1925–2014)

Shulgin is arguably the best known and most highly regarded advocates of so-called designer drugs within the scientific community. He is thought to have synthesized and tested more than 200 psychoactive compounds in his life and wrote a number of important books and articles on the properties and potential benefits of such substances.

Alexander Shulgin, widely known as "Sasha," was born in Berkeley, California, on June 17, 1925. He graduated from high school at the age of sixteen and received a full scholarship to Harvard University. His tenure at Harvard was cut short, however, with the beginning of World War II, during which he served with the U.S. Navy in both the North Atlantic and the Pacific campaigns. After the war, he returned to Berkeley, where he eventually earned his B.A. in chemistry at the University of California in 1949 and his Ph.D. in biochemistry at 1954. He completed his postdoctoral studies at the University of California at San Francisco (UCSF) in pharmacology and psychiatry. After working for a year at the BioRad Laboratories company, he took a position with Dow Chemical, where he was a research scientist from 1955 to 1961 and senior research chemist from 1961 to 1966.

Shulgin's most significant accomplishment at Dow as to develop a pesticide known as physostigmine, a substance that was to become one of Dow's best-selling products. In appreciation of Shulgin's work, Dow provided him with a laboratory of his own where he was allowed to work on projects that were of special interest to him. One of those projects turned out to be the synthesis and study of psychedelic compounds. Shulgin later reported that his interest in psychedelics was prompted by his first experience in taking mescaline in 1960. He told an interviewer from *Playboy* magazine in 2004 that as a result of that experience, he had found his "learning path," the direction he wanted the rest of his career to go.

In 1965, Shulgin decided to leave Dow in order to enter medical school at UCSF. He left that program after only two years, however, to pursue his interest in psychedelics. That decision posed a problem for both Shulgin and the U.S. Drug Enforcement Administration (DEA), the federal agency responsible for control of illegal drug use in the United States. Although their primary function is to discourage the development and use of illegal drugs, the DEA apparently saw some benefit in Shulgin's work, and they agreed to a special dispensation that allowed him to synthesize and study a number of otherwise illegal substances. That relationship eventually worked out well for both partners, as it permitted Shulgin to pursue the studies in which he was most interested and provided the DEA with invaluable information on substances about which they might otherwise have little or no information. In 1988, for example, he wrote *Controlled Substances: Chemical & Legal Guide to Federal Drug Laws*, a book that has become a standard reference for DEA employees.

Shulgin's special relationship with the DEA ended in 1994, when the agency raided his Berkeley laboratory and withdrew his license to conduct research on illegal substances, claiming that he had failed to keep proper records. Some observers believe, however, that the agency's actions were prompted by a book that Shulgin and his wife, Ann, had written a few years earlier: *PiHKAL: A Chemical Love Story*. (*PiHKAL* stands for "phenylethylamines I have known and loved.") The Shulgins later wrote a second book about another group of psychedelic substances: *TiKHAL: The Continuation*. In this case, the word *TiKHAL* stands for "tryptamines I have known and loved." A later Shulgin book was somewhat more technically oriented: *The Simple Plant Isoquinolines* (with Wendy E. Perry). In 2008, his first two laboratory books were scanned and placed online.

Shulgin's health began to decline in 2008 after surgery on a defective aortic valve. He later suffered a strong liver cancer and dementia. He died at his home in Lafayette, California, on June 2, 2014.

Daniel B. Smith (1792–1883)

Smith is remembered today for his role in the creation of the earliest group of pharmaceutical specialists in the United States. He has been called the patriarch of American pharmacy, often grouped with his student and father of American pharmacy William Proctor Jr. Smith, and was among the founders of the first college of pharmacy in the United States, the Philadelphia College of Pharmacy, in 1821, of the first pharmaceutical journal in the United States, the *American Journal of Pharmacy*, in 1826, and of the first professional organization for pharmacists, the American Pharmaceutical Association (now the American Pharmacists Association), in 1852.

Daniel Burlington Smith was born in Philadelphia on July 14, 1792. (Smith appears to have adopted his middle name at some point during his adult life.) His parents were Benjamin and Deborah Smith (née Morris). Benjamin died within a year of Daniel's birth, and his mother decided to return to her hometown of Burlington, New Jersey (perhaps the source of Smith's middle name). Smith received his early education at a Quaker school operated by one John Griscom, also thought to be the first teacher of chemistry in the state of New Jersey. Some record exists of Smith's early interest in ornithology, and his reconstruction of a dead bald eagle drew comment from specialists in the field while he was still a young man. In fact, Smith's combination of pharmaceutical and taxidermical skills has been credited as providing John James Audubon with the paints he used in his highest quality paintings.

Upon completion of his primary education in Burlington, Smith was apprenticed to one John Biddle, an apothecary of some renown in the city of Philadelphia. Smith remained with

Biddle until he was old enough to join his master as a partner. Upon Biddle's death in 1818, Smith opened his own pharmacy in downtown Philadelphia. A decade later, he took one William Hodgson as a partner, forming a company that he continued to operate for most of the rest of his life.

In addition to the professional accomplishments listed here, Smith was active in other fields of pharmacology and in the Philadelphia academic and social communities in general. One of the first of such endeavors dates to 1816, when Smith joined with a group of other Philadelphians to form a financial organization in which tradesmen, mechanics, laborers, house servants, and other workers could deposit and earn interest on their savings. By the end of his life, the Philadelphia Savings Fund had attracted more than 350,000 depositors with total assets of nearly $94 million. Four years later, Smith was one of three founders of a free library for young mechanics and manufacturers. The program was later to develop into the Apprentices' Library Company of Philadelphia, one of the first of its kind in the country.

Yet another of his contributions to the community dates to 1828, when Smith was one of the founders of the House of Refuge for Juvenile Delinquents, an institution created as an alternative to prison for young offenders. Six years later, he was appointed Professor of Moral Philosophy, English Literature, and Chemistry at the Haverford School (now Haverford College) in Philadelphia. He also served as superintendent of the school from 1843 to 1846.

In 1849, Smith decided to withdraw from the very active life to which he had become accustomed and moved to Germantown, Pennsylvania. He died there on March 29, 1883, at the age of 92. In 1965, the American Pharmaceutical Association established the Daniel B. Smith Award for Excellence in the Practice of Pharmacy, a prize that is still issued annually to outstanding members of the profession.

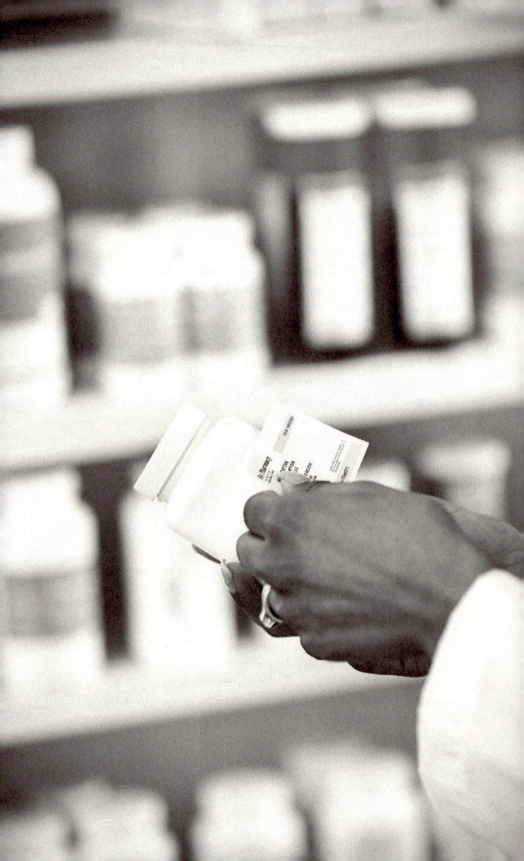

Among the many sources of information available about prescription drugs are data sets and documents relating to the topic. Data sets provide information about the relative popularity, by one standard or another, of most prescription drugs in popular use: the number of drugs used, the prices paid, the demographics of those who use them, the companies that manufacture and sell them, and expected and unexpected consequences of their use are some examples. The data sets provided in the first part of this chapter provide that type of information. In addition, a variety of documents provide an outlook on public and governmental views on the production, sale, use, and effects of such products. These documents include statements by public officials, private citizens, and others; laws and regulations and court cases; and other written statements on the subject. The number of such documents is very large, and the items presented here are no more than examples of the types of official commentaries presented on prescription drugs throughout history.

Data

Questions sometimes arise as to whether drug abuse is primarily an urban or a rural problem. Table 5.1 tracks the relative number and rates of deaths for both settings from 1999 to 2017.

Americans are increasingly interested in finding ways to reduce the cost of prescription drugs they need and buy.

A pharmacist reviews the label on a prescription drug bottle. (sjlockeview/iStockPhoto)

Table 5.1 Urban-Rural Differences in Drug Overdose Death Rates, by Sex, Age, and Type of Drugs Involved, 1999–2017

	Total		Urban		Rural	
Year	Number	Deaths per 100,000	Number	Year	Number	Deaths per 100,000
1999	16,849	60.1	15,120	1999	16,849	60.1
2000	17,415	60.2	15,408	2000	17,415	60.2
2001	19,394	60.8	16,937	2001	19,394	60.8
2002	23,518	8.2	20,512	2002	23,518	8.2
2003	25,785	8.9	22,263	2003	25,785	8.9
2004	27,424	9.4	23,394	2004	27,424	9.4
2005	29,813	10.1	25,520	2005	29,813	10.1
2006	34,425	11.5	29,321	2006	34,425	11.5
2007	36,010	11.9	30,604	2007	36,010	11.9
2008	36,450	11.9	30,862	2008	36,450	11.9
2009	37,004	11.9	31,266	2009	37,004	11.9
2010	38,329	12.3	32,323	2010	38,329	12.3
2011	41,340	13.2	34,853	2011	41,340	13.2
2012	41,502	13.1	35,264	2012	41,502	13.1
2013	43,982	13.8	37,547	2013	43,982	13.8
2014	47,055	14.7	40,272	2014	47,055	14.7
2015	52,404	16.3	45,059	2015	52,404	16.3
2016	63,632	19.8	55,596	2016	63,632	19.8
2017	70,237	21.7	61,712	2017	70,237	21.7

Source: "Data Brief 345: Urban-Rural Differences in Drug Overdose Death Rates, by Sex, Age, and Type of Drugs Involved, 2017." Centers for Disease Control and Prevention. https://www.cdc.gov/nchs/data/databriefs/db345_tables-508.pdf.

Table 5.2 summarizes the three most common methods used to achieve this goal for the period 2013 and 2017.

A common observation about the cost of prescription drugs in the United States points out how much more expensive those drugs are here than in other countries in the world. Table 5.3 summarizes one study of the relative cost of prescription drugs in a dozen countries and the United States.

Many observers have commented on the rapid rise of prescription drug costs in the past decade. Table 5.4 summarizes some of the data on that topic.

Table 5.2 Strategies Used by U.S. Adults to Reduce Cost of Prescription
Drugs, 2013–2017 (Percent of Respondents)

Year	Asked Doctor for Lower-Cost Medication	Did Not Take Medication as Prescribed	Used Alternative Therapies
2013	25.8	14.9	5.8
2014	22.2	12.4	5.2
2015	19.8	11.1	4.8
2016	20.0	10.9	5.2
2017	19.5	11.4	5.4

Source: "Data Brief 333. Strategies Used by Adults Aged 18–64 to Reduce
Their Prescription Drug Costs, 2017." 2019. NCHS Data Brief No. 333. https://
www.cdc.gov/nchs/data/databriefs/db333_tables-508.pdf#page=1.

Table 5.3 Descriptive Statistics on Prescription Drug Prices for Select
Countries, 2018

Country	Average ($)	Minimum ($)	Maximum ($)	Spending per Capita ($)	Number of Drugs
United States	466.15	5.36	16,597.86	1,220.00	79
United Kingdom	105.45	0.08	2,921.09	469.00	78
Japan	69.50	0.15	488.66	838.00	58
Canada (Ontario)	132.59	0.27	3,557.82	832.00	47
Australia	113.57	0.67	3,043.87	673.00	62
Portugal	82.97	0.32	682.02	403.00	37
France	104.51	0.42	2,455.79	653.00	54
Netherlands	152.86	1.42	3,742.87	396.00	61
Germany	165.01	0.46	4,728.76	823.00	65
Denmark	182.29	0.90	4,719.68	318.00	65
Sweden	143.91	0.54	3,612.73	515.00	59
Switzerland	116.22	0.69	3,475.85	963.00	72
Average	152.92	0.08	16,597.86	675.25	79
Average (excluding the United States)	124.45	0.08	4,728.76	625.73	59.9

Source: "A Painful Pill to Swallow: U.S. vs. International Prescription Drug Prices."
2019. Ways and Means Committee Staff, Table 1, page 15. https://waysandmeans.
house.gov/sites/democrats.waysandmeans.house.gov/files/documents/
U.S.%20vs.%20International%20Prescription%20Drug%20Prices_0.pdf.

Table 5.4 Median Total Cost of Top-Selling Brand-Name Drugs, 2012–2017

Brand Name	Treatment or Condition	Median Cost ($)		Six-Year Change (%)
		January 2012	December 2012	
Advair	Chronic obstructive pulmonary disease	225	360	60
Androgel	Testosterone	321	566	76
Atripla	HIV	1776	2531	43
Brilinta	Anticoagulant	236	333	41
Chantix	Smoking cessation	175	392	124
Cialis	Erectile dysfunction	127	365	187
Creon Exocrine	pancreatic insufficiency	293	487	66
Crestor	Cholesterol	146	261	79
Eliquis	Anticoagulant	258	388	50*
Enbrel	Autoimmune disease	1862	4334	133
Farxiga	Type 2 diabetes	318	431	35*
Forteo	Osteoporosis	1116	3088	177
Harvoni	Hepatitis C	31 752	30 920	–3*
Humalog	Insulin	126	274	117
Humira	Autoimmune disease	1940	4338	124
Humulin	Insulin	67	146	117
Invokana	Type 2 diabetes	295	427	58*
Isentress	HIV	1005	1379	37
Januvia	Type 2 diabetes	219	396	80
Lantus	Insulin	212	384	82
Lexapro	Depression	120	300	150
Lipitor	Cholesterol	116	274	137
Lyrica	Pain	174	411	137
Nexium	Gastroesophageal reflux	188	252	34
Novolog	Insulin	244	532	118
Onfi	Seizures	496	996	118*
Orencia	Autoimmune disease	2482	3777	55*
Otezla	Psoriasis	1913	3118	61*
Premarin	Menopause	68	156	129
Prezista	HIV	1119	1454	38*
Pulmicort	Asthma/IBD	151	216	43
Renvela	Kidney disease	212	501	136
Restasis	Immunosuppression	266	463	74

Brand Name	Treatment or Condition	Median Cost ($)		Six-Year Change (%)
		January 2012	December 2012	
Simponi	Autoimmune disease	1978	4094	107
Stelara	Psoriasis	5420	9213	70
Stribild	HIV	2402	3069	28*
Symbicort	Asthma/chronic obstructive pulmonary disease	225	308	37
Synthroid	Thyroid	20	35	72
Tivicay	HIV	1200	1526	28*
Triumeq	HIV	2239	2578	16*
Trulicity	Type 2 diabetes	497	674	35*
Truvada	HIV	1188	1557	31
Viagra	Erectile dysfunction	127	370	190
Victoza	Type 2 diabetes	433	805	86
Viread	HIV	746	1057	42
Vyvanse	Attention deficit hyperactivity disorder	162	270	67
Xarelto	Anticoagulant	225	386	72
Xeljanz	Autoimmune disease	2108	3757	79*
Zetia	Cholesterol	126	313	149

*Drug was not available during the entire study period; the cost indicates the relative price change from first month of claim occurrences (January 2012 entry included data from the first month of occurrence).

Source: Wineinger, Nathan E., Yunyue Zhang, and Eric J. Topol. 2019. "Trends in Prices of Popular Brand-Name Prescription Drugs in the United States." *JAMA Network Open*. 2(5): e194791. doi:10.1001/jamanetworkopen.2019.4791, Table, page 5/9. Used by permission of the authors.

Table 5.5 summarizes the rate of drug use by various populations according to amount of use and over time.

As shown in Table 5.6, the rate of prescription drug use differs substantially among various age groups.

As is to be expected, the type of prescription drug differs according to age group. Table 5.7 summarizes some general information on that topic.

Table 5.5 Prescription Drug Use in the Past 30 Days, by Sex, Race and Hispanic Origin, and Age: United States, Selected Years 1988–1994 through 2013–2016 (Percent of Population)

Trait	At Least One Prescription Drug in Past 30 Days				Three or More Prescription Drugs in Past 30 Days				Five or More Prescription Drugs in Past 30 Days			
	1988–1994	1999–2002	2009–2012	2013–2016	1988–1994	1999–2002	2009–2012	2013–2016	1988–1994	1999–2002	2009–2012	2013–2016
Both sexes	39.1	45.2	47.3	45.8	11.8	17.8	20.6	21.8	4.0	7.5	10.1	11.2
Male	32.7	39.8	42.7	41.7	9.4	14.8	19.1	20.1	2.9	6.1	9.3	10.1
Female	45.0	50.3	51.8	49.7	13.9	20.4	22.0	23.4	4.9	8.7	10.8	12.3
Not Hispanic or Latino												
White only	41.1	48.7	52.4	49.9	12.4	18.9	22.0	23.4	4.2	7.8	10.6	11.8
Male	34.2	43.0	47.2	45.3	9.9	15.9	20.2	21.6	3.1	6.3	9.6	10.6
Female	47.6	54.3	57.6	54.5	14.6	21.8	23.8	25.1	5.1	9.2	11.5	12.9
Black only	36.9	40.1	43.7	44.6	12.6	16.5	21.9	22.4	3.8	7.7	10.9	12.8
Male	31.1	35.4	37.5	40.2	10.2	14.5	19.2	20.0	2.9	6.4	9.5	11.1
Female	41.4	43.8	48.8	48.0	14.3	18.1	24.0	24.3	4.5	8.7	12.0	14.2
Asian only	—	—	—	33.7	—	—	—	14.1	—	—	—	7.1
Male	—	—	—	30.9	—	—	—	14.4	—	—	—	6.5
Female	—	—	—	36.0	—	—	—	14.0	—	—	—	7.6
Hispanic or Latino	--	—	35.4	36.8	—	—	15.9	17.2	—	—	8.4	8.9
Male	—	—	31.7	33.0	—	—	14.7	16.1	—	—	7.8	8.5
Female	—	—	39.2	40.5	—	—	17.1	18.3	—	—	8.9	9.4
Mexican origin	31.7	31.7	34.0	35.1	9.0	11.2	15.4	17.1	2.9	4.4	8.3	9.2
Male	27.5	25.8	30.7	33.1	7.0	9.5	14.0	16.1	2.0	3.5	7.6	8.8
Female	36.0	37.8	37.6	37.3	11.0	12.8	16.8	18.2	3.7	5.2	8.9	9.7

Source: "Prescription Drug Use in the Past 30 Days, by Sex, Race and Hispanic Origin, and Age: United States, Selected Years 1988–1994 through 2013–2016." 2018. Health, United States, 2018—Data Finder. Centers for Disease Control and Prevention. https://www.cdc.gov/nchs/data/hus/2018/038.pdf.

Table 5.6 Trends in Use of One or More Prescription Drugs in the Past 30 Days, by Age, 2007–2016 (Percent)

Survey Period	All Ages	0–11	12–19	20–59	60 and over
2007–2008	48.3	22.4	29.9	48.3	88.4
2009–2010	47.3	23.2	24.7	47.8	86.6
2011–2012	48.0	20.4	29.2	48.7	87.3
2013–2014	46.6	18.0	22.5	48.5	87.1
2015–2016	45.8	18.0	27.0	46.7	85.0

Source: "Trends in Use of One or More Prescription Drugs in the Past 30 Days, by Age (Years): United States, 2007–2016." 2018. Prescription Drug Use in the United States, 2015–2016. Centers for Disease Control and Prevention. https://www.cdc.gov/nchs/data/databriefs/db334_tables-508.pdf#page=4.

Table 5.7 Most Commonly Used Prescription Drug Types in the Past 30 Days, by Age Group, 2015–2016

Age Group (Years) and Drug Type	Percent
0–11	
Penicillins (infections)	2.7
Central nervous system stimulants (attention deficit disorder)	3.5
Bronchodilators (asthma)	4.3
12–19	
Oral contraceptives (birth control, regulate menstruation)	3.7
Bronchodilators (asthma)	3.7
Central nervous system stimulants (attention deficit disorder)	6.2
20–59	
Lipid-lowering drugs (high cholesterol)	7.5
Analgesics (pain relief)	8.3
Antidepressants	11.4
60 and over	
Antidiabetic drugs	22.6
Beta blockers (high blood pressure, heart disease)	24.9
Lipid-lowering drugs (high cholesterol)	46.3

Source: "Most Commonly Used Prescription Drug Types in the Past 30 Days, by Age Group: United States, 2015–2016." Prescription Drug Use in the United States, 2015–2016. Centers for Disease Control and Prevention. https://www.cdc.gov/nchs/data/databriefs/db334_tables-508.pdf#page=4.

DOCUMENTS

Durham-Humphrey Amendment (1951)

This document is an Amendment to the Federal Food, Drug, and Cosmetic Act of 1938, which was the standard federal law for the monitoring and approval of foods and drugs intended for general consumer use. The Durham-Humphrey Amendment resolved three issues that had been left undetermined by the 1938 Act: the definition of prescription drugs, their differences from over-the-counter drugs (OTC), and the mechanism by which the Food and Drug Administration (FDA) was to have control over prescription drugs. A key feature of the Act was inclusion of a mandatory warning on the label of a drug, as indicated in the last paragraph in the following extract. The major sections of this short law are given here.

Be it enacted That subsection (b) of section 503 of the Federal Food, Drug, and Cosmetic Act, as amended, is amended to read as follows:

"(b)(1) A drug intended for use by man which—

"(A) is a habit-forming drug to which section 502 (d) applies;

or

"(B) because of its toxicity or other potentiality for harmful effect, or the method of its use, or the collateral measures necessary to its use, is not safe for use except under the supervision of a practitioner licensed by law to administer such drug; or

"(C) is limited by an effective application under section 505 to use under the professional supervision of a practitioner licensed by law to administer such drug, shall be dispensed only (I) upon a written prescription of a practitioner licensed by law to administer such drug, or (ii) upon an oral prescription of such practitioner which is reduced

promptly to writing and filed by the pharmacist, or (iii) by refilling any such written or oral
prescription if such refilling is authorized by the
prescriber either in the original prescription or by
oral order which is reduced promptly to writing
and filed by the pharmacist. The act of dispensing
a drug contrary to the provisions of this paragraph
shall be deemed to be an act which results in the
drug being misbranded while held for sale.

"(2) Any drug dispensed by filling or refilling a written or oral prescription of a practitioner licensed by
law to administer such drug shall be exempt from
the requirements of section 502, except paragraphs
(a), (I) (2) and (3), (k), and (1), and the packaging
requirements of paragraphs (g) and (h), if the drug
bears a label containing the name and address of the
dispenser, the serial number and date of the prescription or of its filling, the name of the prescriber, and,
if stated in the prescription, the name of the patient,
and the directions for use and cautionary statements,
if any, contained in such prescription. This exemption
shall not apply to any drug dispensed in the course of
the conduct of a business of dispensing drugs pursuant
to diagnosis by mail, or to a drug dispensed in violation of paragraph (1) of this subsection.

"(3) The Administrator may by regulation remove drugs
subject to section 502 (d) and section 505 from the
requirements of paragraph (1) of this subsection when
such requirements are not necessary for the protection
of the public health.

"(4) A drug which is subject to paragraph (1) of this subsection shall be deemed to be misbranded if at any time
prior to dispensing its label fails to bear the statement
"Caution: Federal law prohibits dispensing without
prescription." A drug to which paragraph (1) of this

subsection does not apply shall be deemed to be mis-branded if at any time prior to dispensing its label bears the caution statement quoted in the preceding sentence."

Source: Public Law 215. Chapter 578. 1951. https://www .govinfo.gov/content/pkg/STATUTE-65/pdf/STATUTE -65-Pg648.pdf.

Controlled Substances Act (1970)

The cornerstone of the U.S. government's efforts to control substance abuse is the Controlled Substances Act of 1970, now a part of the U.S. Code, Title 21, Chapter 13. That Act established the system of "schedules" for various categories of drugs that is still used by agencies of the U.S. government today. It also provides extensive background information about the domestic and international status of drug abuse efforts. Some of the most relevant sections for the domestic portion of the Act are reprinted here.

Sections 801 and 801(a) review the competing features of a drug covered by this Act: its possible medical benefits and its potential for misuse.

§ 801. Congressional Findings and Declarations: Controlled Substances

The Congress makes the following findings and declarations:

(1) Many of the drugs included within this subchapter have a useful and legitimate medical purpose and are necessary to maintain the health and general welfare of the American people.

(2) The illegal importation, manufacture, distribution, and possession and improper use of controlled substances have a substantial and detrimental effect on the health and general welfare of the American people.

. . .

§801a. Congressional Findings and Declarations: Psychotropic Substances

The Congress makes the following findings and declarations:

(1) The Congress has long recognized the danger involved in the manufacture, distribution, and use of certain psychotropic substances for nonscientific and nonmedical purposes, and has provided strong and effective legislation to control illicit trafficking and to regulate legitimate uses of psychotropic substances in this country. Abuse of psychotropic substances has become a phenomenon common to many countries, however, and is not confined to national borders. It is, therefore, essential that the United States cooperate with other nations in establishing effective controls over international traffic in such substances.

Section 811 is the key section of this Act. It deals, first of all, with the attorney general's authority for classifying and declassifying drugs and the manner in which these steps are to be taken. In general:

§ 811. Authority and Criteria for Classification of Substances

(a) Rules and Regulations of Attorney General; Hearing

The Attorney General shall apply the provisions of this subchapter to the controlled substances listed in the schedules established by section 812 of this title and to any other drug or other substance added to such schedules under this subchapter. Except as provided in subsections (d) and (e) of this section, the Attorney General may by rule—

(1) add to such a schedule or transfer between such schedules any drug or other substance if he—

    (A) finds that such drug or other substance has a potential for abuse, and

(B) makes with respect to such drug or other substance the findings prescribed by subsection (b) of section 812 of this title for the schedule in which such drug is to be placed; or

(2) remove any drug or other substance from the schedules if he finds that the drug or other substance does not meet the requirements for inclusion in any schedule.

The next section deals with the criteria to be used in determining the status of a drug.

(c) Factors Determinative of Control or Removal from Schedules

In making any finding under subsection (a) of this section or under subsection (b) of section 812 of this title, the Attorney General shall consider the following factors with respect to each drug or other substance proposed to be controlled or removed from the schedules:

(1) Its actual or relative potential for abuse.

(2) Scientific evidence of its pharmacological effect, if known.

(3) The state of current scientific knowledge regarding the drug or other substance.

(4) Its history and current pattern of abuse.

(5) The scope, duration, and significance of abuse.

(6) What, if any, risk there is to the public health.

(7) Its psychic or physiological dependence liability.

(8) Whether the substance is an immediate precursor of a substance already controlled under this subchapter.

Section 812 establishes the Schedules (always capitalized) of drugs covered by this law. Only the details for Schedule I are listed here. Similar descriptions for the other Schedules follow in the text of Section 812.

§ 812. Schedules of Controlled Substances

(a) Establishment

There are established five schedules of controlled substances, to be known as schedules I, II, III, IV, and V. Such schedules shall initially consist of the substances listed in this section. The schedules established by this section shall be updated and republished on a semiannual basis during the two-year period beginning one year after October 27, 1970, and shall be updated and republished on an annual basis thereafter.

(b) Placement on Schedules; Findings Required

Except where control is required by United States obligations under an international treaty, convention, or protocol, in effect on October 27, 1970, and except in the case of an immediate precursor, a drug or other substance may not be placed in any schedule unless the findings required for such schedule are made with respect to such drug or other substance. The findings required for each of the schedules are as follows:

(1) Schedule I.—

   (A) The drug or other substance has a high potential for abuse.

   (B) The drug or other substance has no currently accepted medical use in treatment in the United States.

   (C) There is a lack of accepted safety for use of the drug or other substance under medical supervision.

Source: Title 21 United States Code (USC) Controlled Substances Act. 1970. Diversion Control Division. Drug Enforcement Administration. https://www.deadiversion.usdoj.gov/21cfr/21usc/.

Orphan Drug Act of 1983

The Orphan Drug Act of 1983 was passed as a way of dealing the lack of interest by drug manufacturers in the development of drugs for rare diseases, defined as diseases affecting fewer than 200,000 citizens of the United States. The rationale for the Act is excerpted here. For detailed provisions of the act, see the Source listed later.

(b) The Congress finds that—

   (1) there are many diseases and conditions, such as Huntington's disease, myoclonus, ALS (Lou Gehrig's disease), Tourette syndrome, and muscular dystrophy which affect such small numbers of individuals residing in the United States that the diseases and conditions are considered rare in the United States;

   (2) adequate drugs for many of such diseases and conditions have not been developed;

   (3) drugs for these diseases and conditions are commonly referred to as "orphan drugs";

   (4) because so few individuals are affected by any one rare disease or condition, a pharmaceutical company which develops an orphan drug may reasonably expect the drug to generate relatively small sales in comparison to the cost of developing the drug and consequently to incur a financial loss;

   (5) there is reason to believe that some promising orphan drugs will not be developed unless changes are made in the applicable Federal laws to reduce the costs of developing such drugs and to provide financial incentives to develop such drugs; and

   (6) it is in the public interest to provide such changes and incentives for the development of orphan drugs.

Source: Public Law 97-414. 1983. U.S. Food and Drug Administration. https://www.fda.gov/media/99546/download.

Drug Price Competition and Patent Term Restoration Act (1984)

The Federal Food, Drug, and Cosmetic Act of 1938 provided for the manufacture of generic drugs, to be studied and approved by the FDA through a process known as Abbreviated New Drug Application (ANDA). The principle was that consumers should have the opportunity to purchase drugs pharmacologically equivalent to prescription drugs but at a lower cost. By the early 1980s, however, it became obvious that this goal was not being achieved. Manufacturers of prescription drugs had developed ways of blocking or increasing the difficulty of producing generic versions of their own prescription drugs. In response to that trend, the U.S. Congress in 1948 adopted the Drug Price Competition and Patent Term Restoration Act to make the licensing of generic drugs somewhat easier than it had been in the past. Essentially, the law provided an abbreviated pathway to approval for a drug that was "essentially similar" to a prescription drug already approved by the FDA. Along with this boost for generic drugs, the Act contained some elements that improved the profitability of traditional "innovator" companies, which invented new drugs. The fundamental provisions of the law are as follows:

Title I—Abbreviated New Drug Applications

SEC. 101. Section 505 of the Federal Food, Drug, and Cosmetic Act (21 U.S.C. 355) is amended by redesignating subsection (j) as subsection (k) and inserting after subsection (i) the following:

"(jXI) Any person may file with the Secretary an abbreviated application for the approval of a new drug.

"(2)(A) An abbreviated application for a new drug shall contain—

"(i) information to show that the conditions of use prescribed, recommended, or suggested in the labeling proposed for the new drug have been previously approved for a drug listed under paragraph (6) (hereinafter in this subsection referred to as a "listed drug");

"(ii)(I) if the listed drug referred to in clause (i) has only one active ingredient, information to show that the active ingredient of the new drug is the same as that of the listed drug;

"(II) if the listed drug referred to in clause (i) has more than one active ingredient, information to show that the active ingredients of the new drug are the same as those of the listed drug, or

"(III) if the listed drug referred to in clause (i) has more than one active ingredient and if one of the active ingredients of the new drug is different and the application is filed pursuant to the approval of a petition filed under subparagraph (C), information to show that the other active ingredients of the new drug are the same as the active ingredients of the listed drug, information to show that the different active ingredient is an active ingredient of a listed drug or of a drug which does not meet the requirements of section 201(p), and such other information respecting the different active ingredient with respect to which the petition was filed as the Secretary may require;

"(iii) information to show that the route of administration, the dosage form, and the strength of the new drug are the same as those of the listed drug referred to in clause (i) or, if the route of administration, the dosage form, or the strength of the new drug is different and the application is filed pursuant to the approval of a petition filed under subparagraph (C), such information respecting the route of administration, dosage form, or strength with respect to which the petition was filed as the Secretary may require;

"(iv) information to show that the new drug is bioequivalent to the listed drug referred to in clause (i), except that if the application is filed pursuant to the approval of a petition filed under subparagraph (C), information to show that the active ingredients of the new drug are of the same pharmacological or therapeutic class as those of the listed drug referred to in clause (i) and the new drug can be expected to have the same therapeutic effect as the listed drug when administered to patients for a condition of use referred to in clause (I);

"(v) information to show that the labeling proposed for the new drug is the same as the labeling approved for the listed drug referred to in clause (i) except for changes required because of differences approved under a petition filed under subparagraph (C) or because the new drug and the listed drug are produced or distributed by different manufacturers;

"(vi) the items specified in clauses (B) through (F) of subsection (b)(1);

"(vii) a certification, in the opinion of the applicant and to the best of his knowledge, with respect to each patent which claims the listed drug referred to in clause (i) or which claims a use for such listed drug for which the applicant is seeking approval under this subsection and for which information is required to be filed under subsection (b) or (c)—

"(I) that such patent information has not been filed,

"(II) that such patent has expired,

"(III) of the date on which such patent will expire, or

"(IV) that such patent is invalid or will not be infringed by the manufacture, use, or sale of the new drug for which the application is submitted; and "(viii) if with respect to the listed drug referred to in clause (I) information was filed under subsection (b) or (c) for a method of use patent which does not claim a use for which the applicant is seeking approval under this subsection, a statement that the method of use patent does not claim such a use."

Source: Public Law 98-417-September 24, 1984, 98 Stat. 1585. https://www.govinfo.gov/content/pkg/STATUTE-98/pdf/STATUTE-98-Pg1585.pdf.

Prescription Drug Marketing Act of 1987

One of the ongoing issues of concern in the field of prescription drugs involves the trade of such products in and out of the United States. At a time when the cost of prescription drugs domestically available continues to skyrocket, calls are made for the importation of the same or similar drugs from foreign countries such as Canada. In 1987, the U.S. Congress responded to this problem by adopting the Prescription Drug Manufacturing Act. The rationale and basic provisions of that Act are provided here.

Sec. 2. Findings

The Congress finds the following:

(1) American consumers cannot purchase prescription drugs with the certainty that the products are safe and effective.

(2) The integrity of the distribution system for prescription drugs is insufficient to prevent the introduction and eventual retail sale of substandard, ineffective, or even counterfeit drugs.

(3) The existence and operation of a wholesale submarket, commonly known as the "diversion market", prevents effective control over or even routine knowledge of the true sources of prescription drugs in a significant number of cases.

(4) Large amounts of drugs are being reimported to the United States as American goods returned. These imports are a health and safety risk to American consumers because they may have become subpotent or adulterated during foreign handling and shipping.

(5) The ready market for prescription drug reimports has been the catalyst for a continuing series of frauds against American manufacturers and has provided the cover for the importation of foreign counterfeit drugs.

(6) The existing system of providing drug samples to physicians through manufacturer's representatives has been abused for decades and has resulted in the sale to consumers of misbranded, expired, and adulterated pharmaceuticals.

(7) The bulk resale of below wholesale priced prescription drugs by health care entities, for ultimate sale at retail, helps fuel the diversion market and is an unfair form of competition to wholesalers and retailers that must pay otherwise prevailing market prices.

(8) The effect of these several practices and conditions is to create an unacceptable risk that counterfeit, adulterated, misbranded, subpotent, or expired drugs will be sold to American consumers.

Sec. 3. Reimportation

Section 801 (21 U.S.C. 381) is amended by redesignating subsection (d) as subsection (e) and by inserting after subsection (c) the following:

"(d)(1) Except as provided in paragraph (2), no drug subject to section 503(b) which is manufactured in a State and exported may be imported into the United States unless the drug is imported by the person who manufactured the drug.

"(2) The Secretary may authorize the importation of a drug the importation of which is prohibited by paragraph (1) if the drug is required for emergency medical care."

Sec. 4. Sales Restrictions

Section 503 (21 U.S.C. 353) is amended by adding at the end the following:

"(c)(1) No person may sell, purchase, or trade or offer to sell, purchase, or trade any drug sample. For purposes of this paragraph and subsection (d), the term 'drug sample' means a unit of a drug, subject to subsection (b), which is not intended to be sold and is intended to promote the sale of the drug. Nothing in this paragraph shall subject an officer or executive of a drug manufacturer or distributor to criminal liability solely because of a sale, purchase, trade, or offer to sell, purchase, or trade in violation of this paragraph by other employees of the manufacturer or distributor.

(2) No person may sell, purchase, or trade, offer to sell, purchase, or trade, or counterfeit any coupon. For purposes of this paragraph, the term 'coupon' means a form which may be redeemed, at no cost or at a reduced cost."

Source: PUBLIC LAW 100-293—Apr. 22, 1988 102 Stat. 95. https://www.govinfo.gov/content/pkg/STATUTE-102/pdf/STATUTE-102-Pg95.pdf.

State Doctor Shopping Laws (1990/2011)

As of early 2021, nearly half of the states in the United States had so-called doctor shopping laws. One of the most important ways in which these laws differ from each other is the extent of their coverage. The two examples shown here illustrate the amount of detail contained in two state laws: South Dakota and Connecticut.

South Dakota

22-42-17. Controlled Substances Obtained Concurrently from Different Medical Practitioners—Misdemeanor

Any person who knowingly obtains a controlled substance from a medical practitioner and who knowingly withholds information from that medical practitioner that he has obtained a controlled substance of similar therapeutic use in a concurrent time period from another medical practitioner is guilty of a Class 1 misdemeanor.

Source: SL 1990, Chapter 168. https://sdlegislature.gov/Stat utes/Codified_Laws/DisplayStatute.aspx.

Connecticut

Sec. 21a-266. (Formerly Sec. 19-472). Prohibited acts. (a) No person shall obtain or attempt to obtain a controlled substance or procure or attempt to procure the administration of a controlled substance (1) by fraud, deceit, misrepresentation or subterfuge, or (2) by the forgery or alteration of a prescription or of any written order, or (3) by the concealment of a material fact, or (4) by the use of a false name or the giving of a false address.

(b) Information communicated to a practitioner in an effort unlawfully to procure a controlled substance, or unlawfully to procure the administration of any such substance, shall not be deemed a privileged communication.

(c) No person shall wilfully make a false statement in any prescription, order, report or record required by this part.

(d) No person shall, for the purpose of obtaining a controlled substance, falsely assume the title of, or claim to be, a manufacturer, wholesaler, pharmacist, physician, dentist, veterinarian, podiatrist or other authorized person.

(e) No person shall make or utter any false or forged prescription or false or forged written order.

(f) No person shall affix any false or forged label to a package or receptacle containing controlled substances.

(g) No person shall alter an otherwise valid written order or prescription except upon express authorization of the issuing practitioner.

(h) No person who, in the course of treatment, is supplied with controlled substances or a prescription therefore by one practitioner shall, knowingly, without disclosing such fact, accept during such treatment controlled substances or a prescription therefor from another practitioner with intent to obtain a quantity of controlled substances for abuse of such substances.

(i) The provisions of subsections (a), (d) and (e) shall not apply to manufacturers of controlled substances, or their agents or employees, when such manufacturers or their authorized agents or employees are actually engaged in investigative activities directed toward safeguarding of the manufacturer's trademark, provided prior written approval for such investigative activities is obtained from the Commissioner of Consumer Protection.

Source: Chapter 420b*. Dependency-Producing Drugs. https://www.cga.ct.gov/current/pub/chap_420b.htm#sec_21a-266.

Prescription Drug User Fee Act (1992)

The Prescription Drug User Fee Act (PDUFA) of 1992 was adopted after many years of debate and discussion about the delay in FDA action on the approval of new drugs. The underlying problem was that the FDA had inadequate staffing to permit the agency to make timely decisions on applications of new drugs submitted by pharmaceutical companies. In some cases, the approval process ran for years, costing a drug manufacturer as much as $10 million per year while *they were waiting for FDA action. In 1992, the Congress adopted a new system for assessing pharmaceutical company fees for various aspects of the approval process. The fees collected in this program were designated for very specific purposes, namely the Center for Drug Evaluation and Research and the Center for Biologics Evaluation and Research. The Act contained a provision requiring that the fee schedule and provisions be updated every five years, which has been the case with PDUFA II (1997), PDUFA III (2002), PDUFA IV (2007), PDUFA V (2012), and PDUFA VI (2017). Each Amendment includes updates and other changes to the basic structure of the Act, although that basic structure has remained essentially intact.*

Sec. 102. Findings

The Congress finds that—

(1) prompt approval of safe and effective new drugs is critical to the improvement of the public health so that patients may enjoy the benefits provided by these therapies to treat and prevent illness and disease;

(2) the public health will be served by making additional funds available for the purpose of augmenting the resources of the Food and Drug Administration that are devoted to the process for review of human drug applications; and

(3) the fees authorized by this title will be dedicated toward expediting the review of human drug applications as set forth in the goals identified in the letters of September 14, 1992, and September 21, 1992, from the Commissioner of Food and Drugs to the Chairman of the Energy and Commerce Committee of the House of Representatives and the Chairman of the Labor and Human Resources Committee of the Senate, as set forth at 138 Cong. Rec. H9099–H9100 (daily ed. September 22,1992).

. . .

Sec. 736. Authority to Assess and Use Drug Fees

"(a) TYPES OF FEES.—Beginning in fiscal year 1993, the Secretary shall assess and collect fees in accordance with this section as follows:

"(1) HUMAN DRUG APPLICATION AND SUPPLE-MENT FEE.—

"(A) IN GENERAL.—Each person that submits, on or after September 1, 1992, a human drug application or a supplement shall be subject to a fee as follows:

"(i) A fee established in subsection (b) for a human drug application for which clinical data (other than bioavailability or bioequivalence studies) with respect to safety or effectiveness are required for approval,

"(ii) A fee established in subsection (b) for a human drug application for which clinical data with respect to safety or effectiveness are not required or a supplement for which clinical data (other than bioavailability or bioequivalence studies) with respect to safety or effectiveness are required."

A section follows providing a schedule on which fees must be paid.

"(2) PRESCRIPTION DRUG ESTABLISHMENT FEE. —Each person that—

**(A) owns a prescription drug establishment, at which is manufactured at least 1 prescription drug product which is not the, or not the same as a, product approved under an application filed under section 505(b)(2) or 505(j), and

**(B) after September 1, 1992, had pending before the Secretary a human drug application or supplement, shall be subject to the annual fee established in subsection (b) for each such establishment, payable on or before January 31 of each year.

"(3) PRESCRIPTION DRUG PRODUCT FEE.—

"(A) IN GENERAL.—Except as provided in subparagraph (B), each person—

"(i) who is named as the applicant in a human drug application for a prescription drug product which is listed under section 510, and

"(ii) who, after September 1, 1992, had pending before the Secretary a human drug application or supplement, shall pay for each such prescription drug product the annual fee established in subsection (b). Such fee shall be payable at the time of the first such listing of such product in each calendar year. Such fee shall be paid only once each year for each listed prescription drug product irrespective of the number of times such product is listed under section 510."

Some exceptions to the aforementioned conditions are listed.

(b) FEE AMOUNTS.—

	FY 1993	FY 1994	FY 1995	FY 1996	FY 1997
Drug Application Fee	$100,000	$150,000	$206,000	$217,000	$233,000
Establishment Fee	$60,000	$88,000	$126,000	$133,000	$138,000
Product Fee	$6,000	$9,000	$12,500	$13,000	$14,000

Source: Public Law 102–571. 1992. https://www.govinfo.gov/content/pkg/STATUTE-106/pdf/STATUTE-106-Pg4491.pdf.

Animal Drug Availability Act (1996)

This book has largely not discussed the fact that prescription drugs are available for treatment of domestic, farm, and other animals, just as they are for humans. A fundamental document in the animal drug testing and approval program is the Animal Drug Availability Act of 1996, along with later amendments and clarifying documents. The basic provisions of that Act are provided here. Following that section is a brief summary of the process by which an animal prescription drug is approved by the FDA.

The Animal Drug Availability Act (H.R. 2508) ("ADAA"), signed by the President [George H. W. Bush] on October 9, 1996, amended the Federal Food, Drug, and Cosmetic Act to provide new flexibility to the way FDA regulates new animal drugs and medicated feeds.

The law was intended to increase the number of approved new animal drugs on the market and was supported by FDA's Center for Veterinary Medicine and a coalition of animal industry groups which included manufacturers of animal health products, veterinarians, and livestock producers. ADAA made changes that were intended to benefit the animal health industry and the nation's animals without compromising FDA's mission to protect the public health. The changes introduced by ADAA include:

- amended the definition of substantial evidence of effectiveness, making the process FDA uses to evaluate and approve new animal drugs more flexible. This change eliminated the requirement for field studies and expanded the types of studies that FDA could consider in support of a finding of substantial evidence of effectiveness.
- provided for more interaction between animal drug sponsors and the FDA during the drug development process. The law requires FDA to grant a presubmission conference, if requested by the sponsor, to discuss the drug development

at its earliest stages. The purpose of a presubmission confer- ence is for FDA and the sponsor to agree on the data needed to establish safety and effectiveness, and the types of studies that can be conducted to generate such data.

- provided a procedure for establishing import tolerances for residues of new animal drugs not approved or condition- ally approved for use in the United States but lawfully used in other countries and present in imported, animal-derived food and food products. Import tolerances provide a basis for importing and legally marketing such animal-derived food and food products in the United States.

- created a new category of drugs, "Veterinary Feed Direc- tive Drugs," that allows the approval and use of new animal drugs in animal feed, on a veterinarian's order.

- permitted a range of acceptable/recommended doses to appear on new animal drug product labeling, rather than one optimum dose.

- In addition, the law gives direction to FDA on how to review supplements that seek to add a minor use or minor species indication to an approved application.

Since enactment in 1996, ADAA's provisions have been implemented by FDA in the following regulations:

- 21 CFR § 514.4—Substantial evidence.
- 21 CFR § 514.5—Presubmission conferences.
- 21 CFR § 514.117—Adequate and well-controlled studies.
- 21 CFR § 558.6—Veterinary feed directive drugs.

In addition, a proposed rule regarding import tolerances was published in the Federal Register on January 25, 2012.

Source: "Animal Drug Availability Act of 1996." 2020. U.S. Food and Drug Administration. https://www.fda.gov/animal-veteri nary/guidance-regulations/animal-drug-availability-act-1996.

A Brief Summary of the Drug Approval Process

- The drug sponsor collects information about the safety and effectiveness of a new animal drug. The sponsor may need to conduct studies to get this information. For any studies that are performed, the sponsor analyzes the results.

- Based on the collected information, the drug sponsor decides if there is enough proof that the drug meets the requirements for approval. The sponsor must prove that the drug is safe and effective for a specific use in a specific animal species. If the drug is for food-producing animals (like cows or chickens), the sponsor must also prove that it's safe for people to eat food from treated animals, such as meat, milk, and eggs.

- If the drug sponsor decides the drug meets the requirements for approval, the sponsor submits a New Animal Drug Application (NADA) to CVM. The NADA includes all the information about the drug and the proposed label.

- A team of CVM personnel, including veterinarians, animal scientists, biostatisticians, chemists, microbiologists, pharmacologists, and toxicologists, reviews the NADA. If the center's team agrees with the sponsor's conclusion that the drug is safe and effective when it is used according to the proposed label, CVM approves the NADA and the drug sponsor can legally sell the drug.

A more detailed description of the process follows in the source listed.

Source: "From an Idea to the Marketplace: The Journey of an Animal Drug through the Approval Process." 2019. U.S. Food and Drug Administration. https://www.fda.gov/animal-veteri nary/animal-health-literacy/idea-marketplace-journey-animal-drug-through-approval-process#summary.

Ryan Haight Online Pharmacy Consumer Protection Act of 2008

As a way of dealing with the problem of online sales of prescription drugs without a valid prescription, the U.S. Congress adopted the Ryan Haight Online Pharmacy Consumer Protection Act of 2008. One provision of that Act requires that a consumer have a "valid prescription" in order to purchase a controlled substance online.

(e) Controlled Substances Dispensed by Means of the Internet

(1) No controlled substance that is a prescription drug as determined under the Federal Food, Drug, and Cosmetic Act [21 U.S.C. 301 et seq.] may be delivered, distributed, or dispensed by means of the Internet without a valid prescription.

(2) As used in this subsection:

(A) The term "valid prescription" means a prescription that is issued for a legitimate medical purpose in the usual course of professional practice by—

(i) a practitioner who has conducted at least 1 in-person medical evaluation of the patient; or

(ii) a covering practitioner.

(B) (i) The term "inperson medical evaluation" means a medical evaluation that is conducted with the patient in the physical presence of the practitioner, without regard to whether portions of the evaluation are conducted by other health professionals.

(ii) Nothing in clause (i) shall be construed to imply that 1 in-person medical evaluation demonstrates that a prescription has been issued for a legitimate medical purpose within the usual course of professional practice.

(C) The term "covering practitioner" means, with respect to a patient, a practitioner who conducts a medical evaluation (other than an in-person medical evaluation) at the request of a practitioner who—

(i) has conducted at least 1 inperson medical evaluation of the patient or an evaluation of the patient through the practice of telemedicine, within the previous 24 months; and

(ii) is temporarily unavailable to conduct the evaluation of the patient.

(3) Nothing in this subsection shall apply to—

(A) the delivery, distribution, or dispensing of a controlled substance by a practitioner engaged in the practice of telemedicine; or

(B) the dispensing or selling of a controlled substance pursuant to practices as determined by the Attorney General by regulation, which shall be consistent with effective controls against diversion.

A second provision of the Act calls for the registration of pharmacies that wish to sell prescription drugs on the Internet, as follows:

(f) Research by practitioners; pharmacies; research applications; construction of Article 7 of the Convention on Psychotropic Substances

The Attorney General shall register practitioners (including pharmacies, as distinguished from pharmacists) to dispense, or conduct research with, controlled substances in schedule II, III, IV, or V and shall modify the registrations of pharmacies so registered to authorize them to dispense controlled substances by means of the Internet, if the applicant is authorized to dispense, or conduct research with respect to, controlled substances under the laws of the State in which he practices. The Attorney General may deny an application for such registration or such modification of registration if the Attorney General determines that the issuance of such registration or modification would be inconsistent with the public interest. In determining the public interest, the following factors shall be considered:

(1) The recommendation of the appropriate State licensing board or professional disciplinary authority.

(2) The applicant's experience in dispensing, or conducting research with respect to controlled substances.

(3) The applicant's conviction record under Federal or State laws relating to the manufacture, distribution, or dispensing of controlled substances.

(4) Compliance with applicable State, Federal, or local laws relating to controlled substances.

(5) Such other conduct which may threaten the public health and safety.

Sources: U.S. Code. Title 21—Food and Drugs. Sections 823 and 829, pages 530, 541. http://www.gpo.gov/fdsys/pkg/US CODE-2011-title21/pdf/USCODE-2011-title21-chap13-subchapI-partC-sec823.pdf; http://www.gpo.gov/fdsys/pkg/USCODE-2011-title21/pdf/USCODE-2011-title21-chap13-subchapI-partC-sec829.pdf.

FDA Bad Ad Program (2010)

Health care providers in the United States, along with consumers, are subjected to a barrage of advertising about both prescription and OTC drugs. According to one study, pharmaceutical companies spent an estimated $29.9 billion on advertising of their products in 2016 (https://jamanetwork.com/journals/jama/fullarticle/2720029). The majority of that cost was spent on advertisements to health care providers, with the remainder going to direct-to-consumer advertising. With that flow of money, one question of importance is how accurate the information provided *in that advertising may be. In the United States, laws have been passed to ensure that such advertising is truthful and accurate. The agency responsible for carrying out the provision of that law is The Office of Prescription Drug Promotion (OPDP) of the Food and Drug Administration. One of the primary activities sponsored by the OPDP is the so-called Bad Ad program. The purpose of that program is to help health care providers recognize potentially false and misleading drug advertising. Some of the elements of that program are as follows:*

FDA's Bad Ad Program is an outreach program designed to help healthcare providers recognize potentially false or misleading prescription drug promotion. The program's goal is to raise awareness among healthcare providers including physicians, physician assistants, nurse practitioners, nurses, pharmacists, pharmacy technicians, and trainees about potentially false or misleading prescription drug promotion while also providing them with an easy way to report it to the Agency. The program is run by the Agency's Office of Prescription Drug Promotion (OPDP) in the Center for Drug Evaluation and Research.

. . .

Bad Ad CE Course and Educational Case Studies

Although healthcare providers are frequently exposed to prescription drug promotion, they often have not received education on recognizing false or misleading prescription drug promotion. As part of FDA's Bad Ad Program, OPDP has an online continuing education (CE) and has developed real-life case studies to help bridge this gap for healthcare providers and trainees.

The CE course is a one-hour, self-paced training to help healthcare providers and trainees learn how to recognize and report potentially false or misleading prescription drug promotion to the FDA. It includes modules regarding the Bad Ad Program, the Science of Influence, FDA Oversight of

Prescription Drug Promotion, Common Prescription Drug Promotion Issues, Real-Life Scenarios, and Reporting Potential Drug Promotion Issues. The CE course is accredited for physicians, physician assistants, nurse practitioners, nurses, pharmacists, and pharmacy technicians. It can also be taken by others for a certificate of completion.

The real-life case studies that OPDP has developed are based on actual Warning and Untitled Letters issued by OPDP to companies regarding alleged false or misleading prescription drug promotion. They are designed to be able to be used in a teaching setting. The case studies include the alleged violative promotional material, the Warning or Untitled Letter that was issued, the prescribing information, and a facilitator guide that can be used by an instructor to lead a discussion in a group setting.

Oversight of Prescription Drug Promotion

Prescription Drug Promotion Must

- Not be false or misleading
- Have a balance between efficacy and risk information
- Reveal material facts about the product being promoted, including facts about consequences that may result from use of the drug

What Types of Promotion Does OPDP Regulate?

OPDP regulates prescription drug promotion made by or on behalf of the drug's manufacturer, packer, or distributor, including:

- TV and radio advertisements
- Written or printed prescription drug promotional materials
- Internet based promotion including social media
- Speaker program presentations
- Sales representative presentations

OPDP Does Not Regulate Promotion of

- Over-the-Counter Drugs
- Certain Biological Products
- Medical Devices
- Foods
- Drugs for Animals
- Compounded Drugs
- Cosmetics
- Dietary Supplements

Common Drug Promotion Issues

- Omitting or downplaying of risk
- Overstating the drug's benefits
- Failing to present a "fair balance" of risk and benefit information
- Omitting material facts about the drug
- Making claims that are not appropriately supported
- Misrepresenting data from studies
- Making misleading drug comparisons
- Misbranding an investigational drug

Source: "The Bad Ad Program." 2020. U.S. Food and Drug Administration. https://www.fda.gov/drugs/office-prescription-drug-promotion/bad-ad-program.

United States ex rel. Michael Mullen v. AmerisourceBergen Corporation, et al. (2018)

The prescription drug industry provides many opportunities for individuals and companies to make very large profits by using illegal or unethical practices in the performance of their activities. Awards in the hundreds of millions or billions of dollars for such activities are no longer rare. In the case described here, the AmerisourceBergen Corporation (ABC) agreed to a settlement with the U.S. Department of Justice for several illegal activities involved in the company's purchase, processing, and distribution of drugs used *for cancer treatments. The selection here provides an overview of the types of activities a drug company could make use of to increase their profit on a product. The court's financial award in the case was $625 million.*

1. From October 21, 2001, through January 31, 2014, the ABC Defendants, through MII [Medical Initiatives, Inc.], repackaged the Covered Drugs from their original sterile vials into syringes and distributed those Pre-Filled Syringes to oncology practices and physicians treating vulnerable cancer patients. The ABC Defendants sought to profit from the excess drug product or overfill contained in the original FDA-approved sterile vials. To harvest the overfill, MII broke the sterility of the original sterile vials, pooled the contents, and repackaged the drugs into Pre-Filled Syringes. In so doing, MII created a greater number of Pre-Filled Syringes than the number of vials OSC purchased, which resulted in extra vials that were then sold to customers for profit.

2. From October 21, 2001, through January 31, 2014, the ABC Defendants sold Pre-Filled Syringes to customers. The Pre-Filled Syringes did not have approved New Drug Applications ("NDA") or Biologics License Applications ("BLA") in effect. No NDA or BLA was ever submitted to the FDA for the Pre-Filled Syringes, and the PreFilled Syringes were never covered by an approved NDA or BLA. Furthermore, the ABC Defendants failed to demonstrate to the FDA that the drug vials repackaged into Pre-Filled Syringes were repackaged in a manner that would ensure the safety and efficacy of the drug product. The ABC Defendants did not submit any safety, stability or sterility data to the FDA or any information showing that the Pre-Filled Syringes' container closure system, packaging, or shipping methods would not adversely impact the safety or efficacy of the repackaged drug product. The ABC Defendants did not provide information to the FDA to establish

that the Pre-Filled Syringes were generally recognized as safe and effective.

3. From October 21, 2001 through January 31, 2014, the ABC Defendants' business model was to sell to oncology practices Pre-Filled Syringes of the Covered Drugs that MII repackaged from their original sterile glass vials. To do so, MII staff broke the sterility of the original sterile vials, pooled the contents, and repackaged the drug product into plastic syringes. Some of the Pre-Filled Syringes contained visible particles of unknown origin, which MII sought to filter out before shipment. However, MII did not conduct any tests to confirm that the filtering process removed the foreign particles. The ABC Defendants represented to physician customers that MII's repackaging procedures followed aseptic technique and complied with all applicable laws when, in fact, that was not uniformly the case. On the few occasions when samples of Pre-Filled Syringes were tested for sterility, some of those samples tested positive for bacteria. The ABC Defendants never recalled any Pre-Filled Syringes.

4. From October 21, 2001 through January 31, 2014, the ABC Defendants used overfill and salvaged vials for resale, which caused double-billing for the same vial of drug product. The ABC Defendants' repackaging operation at MII allowed some vials to remain unopened (the "Unopened Vials"). The ABC Defendants resold the Unopened Vials to other healthcare providers. These Unopened Vials were billed to payors, including the Federal healthcare programs. The second purchaser was either another physician ordering vials to be made into Pre-Filled Syringes or a hospital or pharmacy that purchased the Unopened Vials with the representation from the ABC Defendants that the Unopened Vials were purchased directly by the ABC Defendants from the manufacturer and sold directly to the second purchaser. The ABC Defendants failed to disclose

to the second purchasers that the Unopened Vials were extra vials accumulated by MII as a result of the Pre-Filled Syringe Program and billed to payors, including Federal healthcare programs.

5. From June 30, 2005 to January 31, 2014, the ABC Defendants paid kickbacks to physicians to induce them to purchase Procrit® in Pre-Filled Syringes rather than the original vials by providing a rebate to physician-customers who purchased the drug in syringe form. The rebate was disguised on the invoice as a general pharmacy credit and not associated with Procrit®. Customers who bought Procrit® in a vial rather than Pre-Filled Syringes did not receive the additional rebate. The ABC Defendants did not properly disclose the rebate to customers in writing at the time of the initial sale of Procrit®.

Source: "Settlement Agreement." 2018. https://www.justice .gov/usao-edny/press-release/file/1097506/download.

American Patients First (2018)

The cost of prescription drugs has long been an issue of concern to both federal and state governments. So far, few entities have had success in finding ways of dealing with this problem. In 2018, President Donald Trump proposed a new plan, American Patients First, that contained the elements that he and his administration believed could reduce the cost of prescription drugs for patients. The following is a summary of that program.

"One of my greatest priorities is to reduce the price of prescription drugs. In many other countries, these drugs cost far less than what we pay in the United States. That is why I have directed my Administration to make fixing the injustice of high drug prices one of our top priorities. Prices will come down."

. . .

HHS [U.S. Department of Health and Human Services] has identified four challenges in the American drug market:

- High list prices for drugs
- Seniors and government programs overpaying for drugs due to lack of the latest negotiation tools
- High and rising out-of-pocket costs for consumers
- Foreign governments free-riding of American investment in innovation

Under President Trump, HHS has proposed a comprehensive blueprint for addressing these challenges, identifying four key strategies for reform:

- Improved competition
- Better negotiation
- Incentives for lower list prices
- Lowering out-of-pocket costs

HHS's blueprint encompasses two phases: (1) actions the President may direct HHS to take immediately and (2) actions HHS is actively considering, on which feedback is being solicited.

Increased Competition
Immediate Actions
- Steps to prevent manufacturer gaming of regulatory processes such as Risk Evaluation and Mitigation Strategies (REMS)
- Measures to promote innovation and competition for biologics
- Developing proposals to stop Medicaid and Affordable Care Act programs from raising prices in the private market

Further Opportunities

- Considering how to encourage sharing of samples needed for generic drug development
- Additional efforts to promote the use of biosimilars

Better Negotiation
Immediate Actions

- Experimenting with value-based purchasing in federal programs
- Allowing more substitution in Medicare Part D to address price increases for single-source generics
- Reforming Medicare Part D to give plan sponsors significantly more power when negotiating with manufacturers
- Sending a report to the President on whether lower prices on some Medicare Part B drugs could be negotiated for by Part D plans
- Leveraging the Competitive Acquisition Program in Part B.
- Working across the Administration to assess the problem of foreign free-riding

Further Opportunities

- Considering further use of value-based purchasing in federal programs, including indication-based pricing and long-term financing
- Removing government impediments to value-based purchasing by private payers
- Requiring site neutrality in payment
- Evaluating the accuracy and usefulness of current national drug spending data

Incentives for Lower List Prices
Immediate Actions

- FDA evaluation of requiring manufacturers to include list prices in advertising

- Updating Medicare's drug-pricing dashboard to make price increases and generic competition more transparent

Further Opportunities

- Measures to restrict the use of rebates, including revisiting the safe harbor under the Anti-Kickback statute for drug rebates
- Additional reforms to the rebating system
- Using incentives to discourage manufacturer price increases for drugs used in Part B and Part D
- Considering fiduciary status for PBMs
- Reforms to the Medicaid Drug Rebate Program
- Reforms to the 340B drug discount program
- Considering changes to HHS regulations regarding drug copay discount cards

Source: "American Patients First: The Trump Administration Blueprint to Lower Drug Prices and Reduce Out-of-Pocket Costs." 2018. U.S. Department of Health and Human Services. https://www.hhs.gov/sites/default/files/AmericanPatientsFirst.pdf.

Generic Drugs: Questions & Answers (2018)

One question that consumers often ask is whether it is safe to use generic drugs. Are they to be trusted to the same extent as are brand-name drugs? The following selection explains how the U.S. FDA decides whether a generic drug meets the standards required to grant it approval.

What Standards Must Generic Medicines Meet to Receive FDA Approval?

Drug companies can submit an abbreviated new drug application (ANDA) for approval to market a generic drug that is the same as (or bioequivalent to) the brand-name version. FDA's

Office of Generic Drugs reviews the application to make certain drug companies have demonstrated that the generic medicine can be substituted for the brand-name medicine that it copies.

An ANDA must show the generic medicine is equivalent to the brand in the following ways:

- The active ingredient is the same as that of the brand-name drug/innovator drug.
  - An active ingredient in a medicine is the component that makes it pharmaceutically active—effective against the illness or condition it is treating.
  - Generic drug companies must provide evidence that shows that their active ingredient is the same as that of the brand-name medicine they copy, and FDA must review that evidence.
- The generic medicine is the same strength.
- The medicine is the same type of product (such as a tablet or an injectable).
- The medicine has the same route of administration (such as oral or topical).
- It has the same use indications.
- The inactive ingredients of the medicine are acceptable.
  - Some differences, which must be shown to have no effect on how the medicine functions, are allowed between the generic and the brand-name version.
  - Generic drug companies must submit evidence that all the ingredients used in their products are acceptable, and FDA must review that evidence.
- It lasts for at least the same amount of time.
  - Most medicines break down, or deteriorate, over time.
  - Generic drug companies must do months-long "stability tests" to show that their versions last for at least the same amount of time as the brand-name.

- It is manufactured under the same strict standards as the brand-name medicine.
  - It meets the same batch requirements for identity, strength, purity, and quality.
  - The manufacturer is capable of making the medicine correctly and consistently.
    - Generic drug manufacturers must explain how they intend to manufacture the medicine and must provide evidence that each step of the manufacturing process will produce the same result each time. FDA scientists review those procedures, and FDA inspectors go to the generic drug manufacturer's facility to verify that the manufacturer is capable of making the medicine consistently and to check that the information the manufacturer has submitted to FDA is accurate.
    - Often, different companies are involved (such as one company manufacturing the active ingredient and another company manufacturing the finished medicine). Generic drug manufacturers must produce batches of the medicines they want to market and provide information about the manufacturing of those batches for FDA to review.
- The container in which the medicine will be shipped and sold is appropriate.
- The label is the same as the brand-name medicine's label.
  - The drug information label for the generic medicine should be the same as the brand-name label. One exception is if the brand-name drug is approved for more than one use and that use is protected by patents or exclusivities. A generic medicine can omit the protected use from its labeling and only be approved for a use that is not protected by patents or exclusivities, so long as that removal does not take away information needed for safe use. Labels for generic medicines can also contain certain

changes when the drug is manufactured by a different company, such as a different lot number or company name.

- Relevant patents or exclusivities are addressed.
  - As an incentive to develop new medicines, drug companies are awarded patents and exclusivities that may delay FDA approval of applications for generic medicines. FDA must comply with the delays in approval that the patents and exclusivities impose.

The ANDA process does not, however, require the drug applicant to repeat costly animal and clinical research on ingredients or dosage forms already approved for safety and effectiveness. This allows generic medicines to be brought to market more quickly and at lower cost, allowing for increased access to medications by the public.

Source: "Generic Drugs: Questions & Answers." 2018. U.S. Food and Drug Administration. https://www.fda.gov/drugs/questions-answers/generic-drugs-questions-answers#q5.

Association for Accessible Medicines v. Frosh (2018)

In 2017, the Maryland General Assembly passed a law designed to reduce the growing cost of drugs in the state. The law applied to generic drugs for which manufacturers had raised prices in a manner deemed to be "unconscionable." It allowed the state attorney general to sue companies that had raised the price of a drug more than 50 percent in one year, without a valid reason for having taken this action. The text of that bill is available at https:// legiscan.com/MD/text/HB631/2017. This action was contested by a professional organization, the Association for Accessible Medicine (AAM), on the basis of the doctrine of Dormant Commerce Clause. That clause arises from the First Amendment of the U.S. Constitution and is designed to prohibit a state legislature from discriminating against interstate or international commerce. In the first trial, a district court rejected the AAM's argument and found in favor of the defendant's, the Maryland House. Upon appeal to the U.S. Court of Appeals for the Fourth Circuit, however, the district court's decision was reversed, and the AAM argument was accepted. The U.S. Supreme Court eventually declined to hear an appeal from this decision, and the Maryland legislation was deemed unconstitutional. The bases for this decision from the appeals court were as follows. Footnotes in the decision have been omitted.

The Association for Accessible Medicines ("AAM") appeals the district court's dismissal of its dormant commerce clause challenge to a Maryland statute prohibiting price gouging in the sale of prescription drugs. AAM also appeals the district court's refusal to enjoin enforcement of the statute on the basis that it is unconstitutionally vague. We hold that the statute violates the dormant commerce clause because it directly regulates the price of transactions that occur outside Maryland. Accordingly, we reverse the district court's dismissal of that claim and remand with instructions to enter judgment in favor of AAM.

. . .

We agree with AAM that the district court erroneously upheld the Act under the dormant commerce clause. First, the Act is not triggered by any conduct that takes place within Maryland. Second, even if it were, the Act controls the prices of transactions that occur outside the state. Finally, the Act, if similarly enacted by other states, would impose a significant burden on interstate commerce involving prescription drugs. All of these factors combine to create a violation of the dormant commerce clause.

. . .

The Act Is Not Limited to Sales Wholly within Maryland

. . .

Therefore, the Act targets conduct that occurs entirely outside Maryland's borders, a conclusion supported by the Act's prohibition of a manufacturer's use of the defense that it did not directly sell to a consumer in Maryland. . . . The district court thus erred in relying on the Act's "made available for sale" language to uphold the Act.

. . .

The Act Impacts Transactions That Occur Wholly Outside Maryland

. . .

Even if the Act did require a nexus to an actual sale in Maryland, it is nonetheless invalid because it still controls the price of transactions that occur wholly outside the state. . . . The Act, by its own terms, is not fixated on the price the Maryland consumer ultimately pays for the drug. Instead, the lawfulness of a price increase is measured according to the price the manufacturer or wholesaler charges in the initial sale of the drug.

. . .

The Act Implicates a Price Control as Opposed to an Upstream Pricing Impact

Therefore, the fundamental problem with the Act is that it "regulate[s] the price of [an] out-of-state transaction." . . . The Act instructs prescription drug manufacturers that they are prohibited from charging an "unconscionable" price in the initial sale of a drug, which occurs outside Maryland's borders. Maryland cannot, even in an effort to protect its consumers from skyrocketing prescription drug costs, impose its preferences in this manner. The "practical effect" of the Act, much like the effect of the statutes struck down in Brown-Forman and Healy, is to specify the price at which goods may be sold beyond Maryland's borders. . . . The district court erred by failing to account for this impact.

The Act Burdens Interstate Commerce in Prescription Drugs

The Act's significant scope is further illuminated by the burden similar legislation would place on interstate commerce. . . .

Because the Act targets wholesale rather than retail pricing, an analogous restriction imposed by a state other than Maryland has the potential to subject prescription drug manufacturers to conflicting state requirements. . . . And the Act's relatively subjective definition of what constitutes an unlawful price increase only exacerbates the problem. If multiple states enacted this type of legislation, then a manufacturer may consummate a transaction in a state where the transaction is fully permissible, yet still be subject to an enforcement action in another state (such as Maryland) wholly unrelated to the transaction.

. . .

In sum, we hold that the Act is unconstitutional under the dormant commerce clause because it directly regulates transactions that take place outside Maryland. We therefore reverse the district court's dismissal of this claim and remand this matter to the district court with instructions to enter judgment in favor of AAM.

To be clear, we in no way mean to suggest that Maryland and other states cannot enact legislation meant to secure lower prescription drug prices for their citizens. Indeed, the Supreme Court upheld a Maine law with that very aim in Walsh.

Although we sympathize with the consumers affected by the prescription drug manufacturers' conduct and with Maryland's efforts to curtail prescription drug price gouging, we are constrained to apply the dormant commerce clause to the Act. Our dissenting colleague suggests that by doing so, we imply that prescription drug manufacturers have a constitutional right to engage in price gouging. This is a sweeping and incorrect conclusion to draw from our holding that Maryland is prohibited from combating prescription drug price gouging in the manner utilized by the Act. Prescription drug manufacturers are by no means "constitutionally entitled," to engage in abusive prescription drug pricing practices. But Maryland must address this concern via a statute that complies with the dormant commerce clause of the U.S. Constitution.

Source: *Association for Accessible Medicines v. Brian E. Frosh and Dennis R. Schrader*. 2018. United States Court of Appeals for the Fourth Circuit. No. 17-2166. https://www.nashp.org/wp-content/uploads/2018/06/AAM-v-Frosh-CA4-Opinion-Reversing-District-Court-April-13-2018.pdf.

Medicare Prescription Drug Coverage (2020)

On July 30, 1965, President Lyndon Johnson signed into law a bill creating the Medicare and Medicaid programs that were to become the basis by which all citizens of the United States were to receive coverage for their health needs when they reached the age of sixty-five. That bill made no provision, however, for coverage of an individual's prescription drug costs. In fact, it took another thirty-eight years before such coverage was included in the Medicare program. In that year, 2003, the U.S. Congress adopted the Medicare Prescription Drug, Improvement, and Modernization Act of 2003, which created Part D of the Medicare program, providing for help in paying one's prescription drug costs. That program has become a complex, but essential, part of every American's health care program. The following section contains some of the main features of Part D coverage.

Medicare Prescription Drug Coverage Adds to Your Medicare Health Coverage

Medicare prescription drug coverage (Part D) helps you pay for both brand-name and generic drugs. Medicare drug plans are offered by insurance companies and other private companies approved by Medicare.

You can get coverage 2 ways:

1. Medicare Prescription Drug Plans (sometimes called "PDPs") add prescription drug coverage to Original Medicare, some Medicare Private Fee-for-Service (PFFS) Plans,

some Medicare Cost Plans, and Medicare Medical Savings Account (MSA) Plans.

2. Some Medicare Advantage Plans (like HMOs or PPOs) or other Medicare health plans offer prescription drug coverage. You generally get all of your Medicare Part A (Hospital Insurance), Medicare Part B (Medical Insurance), and Part D through these plans. Medicare Advantage Plans that offer prescription drug coverage are sometimes called "MA-PDs."

. . .

How Much Will My Drug Coverage Cost?

Medicare drug plans have different coverage and costs, but all must offer at least a standard level of coverage set by Medicare. How much you actually pay for Medicare drug coverage depends on which drugs you use, which Medicare drug plan you join, whether you go to a pharmacy in your plan's network, and whether you get Extra Help paying for your drug costs. Contact the plan(s) you're interested in to get specific cost information.

Your drug coverage costs are affected by:

- Monthly premium
- Yearly deductible
- Copayments or coinsurance
- Coverage gap (also called the "donut hole")
- Catastrophic coverage

Monthly Premium

Most drug plans charge a monthly fee that differs from plan to plan. You pay this fee in addition to the Part B premium. If you belong to a Medicare Advantage Plan (like an HMO or PPO) or a Medicare Cost Plan that includes Medicare drug coverage, the monthly premium may include an amount for drug coverage.

Some people with Medicare may pay a higher monthly premium based on their income. If you reported a modified adjusted gross income of more than $85,000 (individuals and married individuals filing separately) or $170,000 (married individuals filing jointly) on your 2017 IRS tax return (the most recent tax return information provided to Social Security by the IRS), you'll have to pay an extra amount for your Medicare drug coverage, called the income-related monthly adjustment amount (IRMAA). You'll pay this extra amount in addition to your monthly Part D plan premium.

Social Security will send you a letter if you have to pay for this extra amount.

. . .

Your adjustment amount will get taken out of your monthly Social Security, Railroad Retirement, or Office of Personnel Management check, no matter how you usually pay your plan premium. If that amount is more than what's in your check, you'll get a bill from Medicare each month.

If you don't pay your entire Part D premium (and the extra amount), you may be disenrolled from your Part D plan. You must pay both the extra amount and your plan's premium each month to keep Medicare drug coverage.

If you have to pay a higher amount for your Part D premium and you disagree, visit socialsecurity.gov, or call 1-800-772-1213. TTY users can call 1-800-325-0778.

Yearly deductible The deductible is what you pay for your drugs before your plan begins to pay. No Medicare drug plan may have a deductible more than $435 in 2020. Some plans don't charge a deductible.

Copayments or Coinsurance

You pay copayments or coinsurance for your drugs after you pay the deductible. You pay your share, and your plan pays its share for covered drugs.

Usually, the amount you pay for a covered drug is for a one-month supply of a drug. However, you can request less than a one-month supply for most types of drugs. You might do this if you're trying a new medication that's known to have significant side effects or you want to get the refills for all your drugs on the same refill schedule. If you do this, the amount you pay is reduced based on the quantity you actually get. Talk with your prescriber (a health care provider who's legally allowed to write prescriptions) to get a drug for less than a one-month supply.

Coverage Gap (also Called the "Donut Hole")

A gradual closing of the coverage gap has made Medicare drug coverage more reasonably priced for people with Medicare. You reach the coverage gap after you and your plan have spent a certain amount of money for covered drugs. When you're in the coverage gap, you may pay more costs for your drugs out-of-pocket, up to a limit.

Not everyone will reach the coverage gap. Your yearly deductible, coinsurance or copayments, and what you pay in the coverage gap all count toward this out-of-pocket limit. The limit doesn't include the drug plan's premium or what you pay for drugs that aren't on your plan's formulary (drug list).

You won't need to pay all out-of-pocket costs when you're in the coverage gap. In 2020, your plan will cover at least 5% of the cost of covered brand-name drugs, and the drug manufacturer will give a 70% discount, for a combined savings of at least 75% on these brand-name drugs. The amount you pay (25%) and the 70% discount you get from the manufacturer both count as out-of-pocket spending that will help you get out of the coverage gap. Also, in 2020, Medicare will cover 75% of the price for generic drugs when you're in the coverage gap.

In 2020, you'll only pay 25% for both covered generic and brand-name drugs when in the gap.

For each month that you fill a prescription, your drug plan mails you an "Explanation of Benefits" (EOB) notice, which tells you how much you've spent on covered drugs and if you've reached the coverage gap. In 2020, your EOB notice will also show the 5% your plan pays and the 70% discount from the drug manufacturer on covered brand-name drugs you buy in the coverage gap.

Source: "Your Guide to Medicare Prescription Drug Coverage." n.d. Centers for Medicare and Medicaid Services. https://www.medicare.gov/Pubs/pdf/11109-Your-Guide-to-Medicare-Prescrip-Drug-Cov.pdf.

The American Hospital Association v. Azar (2020)

In his decision, Judge Carl Nichols writes that "the impenetrability of hospital bills is legendary." He goes on to call hospital billing as "arcane" and "mystifying" (p. 2). The case before the judge was a suit filed by the American Hospital Association and other hospital groups (the plaintiffs) challenging a new set of rules dealing with transparency in pricing of hospital services. That rule can be found in its entirety at https://www.hhs.gov/sites/default/files/cms-1717-f2.pdf. The purpose of the rule was to make it easier for American consumers to understand the charges they may be levied for services at a hospital. In the case filed by the plaintiffs, the judge found for the defendants, rejecting the numerous specific complaints raised by the plaintiffs. The decision was of some importance to the issue of health care cost transparency in general and also because of the pending—at the time of the ruling—rule on transparency in health care coverage affecting insurance and related companies. Salient portions of Judge Nichols's decision are as follows. (References have been omitted.)

Plaintiffs do not appear to dispute that the agency's asserted interest in increasing transparency is substantial. Instead, they argue that the Rule is unjustified because the publication of hundreds of prices will "confuse" patients and "frustrate. . . [their] deci-sionmaking." . . . They further contend that the regulation is unduly burdensome. . . . The agency has explained it has two interests: "providing consumers with factual price information to facilitate more informed health care decisions" and "lower-ing healthcare costs." . . . According to the agency, publications of the five types of charges advances those interests. Patients want to make informed choices, but the lack of price transpar-ency is one of the biggest hurdles they face in navigating the health care market to find the best value. . . . Case studies from various states have shown that where patients have access to pricing information, they can and will use price transparency tools to inform their health care choices. . . . Consumers in New Hampshire and Maine, which have required the publica-tion of select negotiated charges, have used pricing informa-tion to their benefit, which has created downward pressure on health care costs. . . . Research suggests that greater price trans-parency, "when available to the entire market," can also reduce health care costs. . . . And access to pricing information allows patients and doctors to have the "cost-of-care conversations at the point of care." . . . The publication of charges will allow the agency to further its interest of informing patients about the cost of care, which will in turn advance its other interest—bringing down the cost of health care.

While it is true that the published charges may not be the out-of-pocket costs for all patients, this does not mean that the disclosures are so incomplete that they are no longer "purely factual and uncontroversial." . . . Even Central Hudson recog-nizes that although some disclosures "communicate . . . only incomplete version of the relevant facts, the First Amend-ment presumes that some accurate information is better than no information at all." . . . Plaintiffs do not meaningfully dis-pute that for some patients, such as those on high deductible health plans, the data will provide at least a useful estimate of the expense of certain hospital services, if not their actual out-of-pocket rates. It may be that those patients will sometimes have to take additional steps to determine their out-of-pocket costs, but unlike chargemaster rates, this information will allow patients to make those calculations. Even where patients may be unable to compute their health costs on their own, various developers have created platforms that aggregate pricing information to let consumers conduct price searches. . . . And more generally, all of the information required to be published by the Final Rule can allow patients to make pricing comparisons between hospitals. . . .

Plaintiffs argue that requiring insurers to publish patients' out-of-pocket costs would be more useful to patients and point to an ongoing rulemaking that would require just that. But Zauderer (like Central Hudson) does not require a perfect fit, only a reasonable one. Plaintiffs also ignore that the Rule enables patients to compare discounted cash prices with negotiated rates to determine which option is the most affordable. . . . Requiring insurance companies to publish patients' out-of-pocket rates does not further the agency's goals of empowering patients in precisely the same way. And, as discussed further below, price transparency advances the government's other interest—lowering health care costs.

Plaintiffs focus on the logistical and financial burdens of compliance with the Rule. But the question of whether a regulation is "unduly burdensome" looks to whether *speech* is burdened or chilled. . . .

Plaintiffs argue that the publication of payer-specific negotiated rates will chill negotiations between hospitals and insurers. . . . But the Rule requires only the publication of the final agreed-upon price—which is also provided to each patient in the insurance-provided explanation of benefits—and not any information about the negotiations themselves. Plaintiffs are essentially attacking transparency measures generally, which are intended to enable consumers to make informed decisions; naturally, once consumers have certain information, their purchasing habits may change, and suppliers of items and services may have to adapt accordingly. (This was implicit in AMI, which recognized that consumers wanted country-of-origin labels and that the mandate was spurred in part by "buy American" interests. . . . Hospitals may be affected by market changes and need to respond to a market where consumers are more empowered, but the possibility that the nature of their negotiations with insurers might change is too attenuated from the compelled disclosure to make the Rule unlawful under Zauderer. And although Plaintiffs assert that the Rule threatens to shut down negotiations altogether, . . . this is contradicted by their arguments implying that negotiations would continue but ultimately benefit insurers.

Source: *The American Hospital Association v. Azar*. Civil Action No. 2019-3619 (D.D.C. 2020). https://ecf.dcd.uscourts.gov/cgi-bin/show_public_doc.

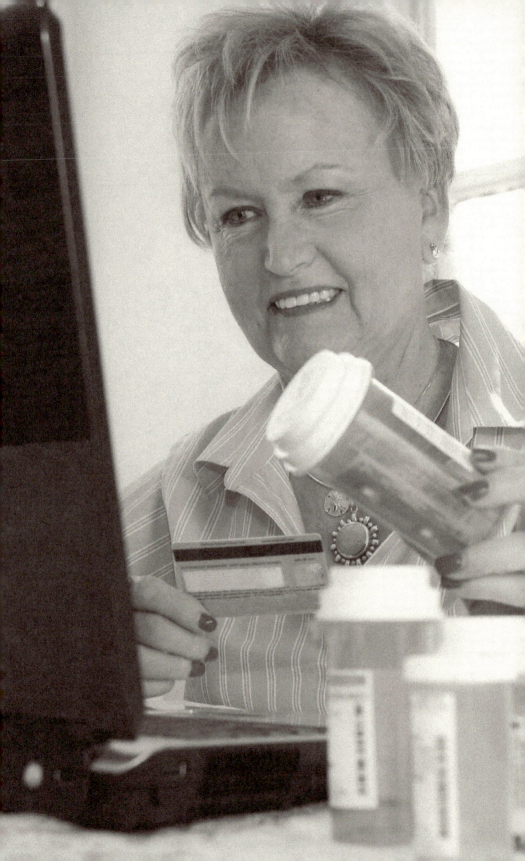

The topic of prescription drugs is one that has been written about in books, articles, reports, and electronic sources for many years. These sources are an invaluable aid to anyone wishes to learn more about a topic or to continue one's own research on the topic. The items listed here are only a sample of the many items available on the subject, but they provide a good overview of the type of information available on the topic. In several instances, an item may be available in more than one form, most commonly as a print article and electronic document. Notations for each item of this kind are provided in the annotation. The reader is advised to recall that the references found at the end of Chapters 1 and 2 are also a good source of further information on the topic of prescription drugs.

Books

Beasley, Henry. 1865. *The Book of Prescriptions Containing 3000 Prescriptions . . . Also, a Compendious History of the Materia Medica, Lists of the Doses of All Officinal or Established Preparations, and an Index of Diseases and Remedies*. Philadelphia: Lindsay.

For those readers interested in the history of prescription concoctions, this book provides a fascinating review of most of the substances in use by pharmacists and other healers in the mid-nineteenth century.

A senior citizen purchases prescription medication online. (Mary Katherine Wynn/Dreamstime.com)

Bell, Edward A. 2017. *Children's Medicines: What Every Parent, Grandparent, and Teacher Needs to Know.* Baltimore: Johns Hopkins Press.

> Protocols for prescribing and administering medicine to children are different in some important ways from those for adults. This book, from the *Johns Hopkins Press Health* series, reviews factors to be considered in the safe and effective use of prescription and nonprescription drugs for children and young adults.

Brownstein, Henry H. 2017. *The Handbook of Drugs and Society.* Hoboken, NJ: Wiley Blackwell.

> The author focuses primarily on the role that drugs play in society, with sections on the use and marketing of particular drugs in society, explaining the place of drugs in society, what we know and do not know about drugs and public health and safety, drugs and adverse social experiences, and drugs as an illicit enterprise.

Bryant, Robert L., and Howard L. Forman. 2019. *Prescription Drug Abuse.* Santa Barbara, CA: Greenwood, an imprint of ABC-CLIO.

> This book, designed especially for young adults, provides all of the basic information one needs to learn more about and continue one's own research on the topic of prescription drug abuse. Chapters One and Two provide a good general introduction to the topic, including data on the problem, current issues in the field, and some of the solutions that have been proposed for dealing with prescription drug abuse. The final section of the book provides some useful resource materials for learning more about the topic.

Chasin, Alexandria. 2016. *Assassin of Youth: A Kaleidoscopic History of Harry J. Anslinger's War on Drugs.* Chicago: The University of Chicago Press.

Although probably not well known today, Anslinger had one of the most significant influences on legal restraints on narcotics in American history. This book provides an excellent overview of his life and his program for drastically restricting the use of opium, cocaine, marijuana, and other psychoactive drugs.

Chen, Keji. 1996. *Imperial Medicaments: Medical Prescriptions Written for Empress Dowager Cixi and Emperor Guangxu with Commentary.* Beijing: Foreign Languages Press.
This volume contains prescriptions for 391 herbal mixtures prepared especially for these early nineteenth-century Chinese rulers. A book of some historical interest for those interested in the development of prescriptions.

Dowling, Harry Filmore. 1970. *Medicines for Man: The Development, Regulation, and Use of Prescription Drugs.* New York: Knopf.
As a former practicing physician, researcher, and medical educator, the author has the broad background needed to provide an incisive look at the development of prescription drugs to the book's publication date.

Dusenbery, Maya. 2018. *Doing Harm: The Truth about How Bad Medicine and Lazy Science Leave Women Dismissed, Misdiagnosed, and Sick.* New York: HarperOne.
One of the neglected problems in both prescription drug policy and practice, as well as health care in general, is the lack of equal attention given to women's issues, compared to men's issues. The author examines the basic reasons for this condition, how it manifests in the use of medicines today, and steps that can be taken to remedy the problem.

Eyre, Eric. 2020. *Death in Mud Lick: A Coal Country Fight against the Drug Companies That Delivered the Opioid Epidemic.* New York: Scribner.

This book is based on the discovery that a small pharmacy in the town of Kermit, West Virginia, filled 12 million prescriptions for opioids in a community of 382 people. The book traces the ways in which the pharmaceutical industry used this practice to feed the nation's opioid abuse epidemic of the 2010s and beyond.

Feldman, Robin, and Evan Frondorf. 2017. *Drug Wars: How Big Pharma Raises Prices and Keeps Generics Off the Market.* New York: Cambridge University Press.

The purpose of this book, according to its authors, is "the schemes, strategies, and tactics—not competition, not R&D—that pharmaceutical companies use to keep prices high and generic drugs off the market, denying consumers billions in cost savings and health benefits each year."

Flanigan, Jessica. 2017. *Pharmaceutical Freedom: Why Patients Have a Right to Self-Medicate.* New York: Oxford University Press.

The author makes the intriguing argument that society exerts unreasonably powerful control over the way prescription drugs are made available to the general public and that individuals should have the right to choose and use any approved drug as they care to do so.

Fust, Kristin, ed. 2019. *Gale Encyclopedia of Prescription Drugs.* 2 vols. Farmington Hills, MI: Gale, Cengage Learning.

This two-volume work is an invaluable, readily accessible guide to more than 300 commonly prescribed drugs, providing information on their normal applications, potential side effects, drug and food interactions, recommended dosages, and warnings and precautions.

Gibson, Rosemary, and Janardan Prasad Singh. 2018. *China Rx: Exposing the Risks of America's Dependence on China for Medicine.* Amherst, NY: Prometheus Books.

The authors point out that millions of Americans routinely depend on prescription drugs manufactured in China. Two major problems are associated with that fact. First, the United States should not depend on any one country for such a large supply of the its need for medications; second, lapses in manufacturing procedures in China tend to result in problems of safety and efficacy of drugs produced in that country.

Hoffman, Daniel, and Allan Bowditch. 2020. *The Global Pharmaceutical Industry: The Demise and the Path to Recovery*. New York: Routledge.
The authors explain that drug companies have been experiencing exorbitant profits, largely through the sale of prescription drugs to "the world's most vulnerable populations." They suggest that national governments have begun to develop punishing legislation to bring this practice under control, and they offer some suggestions for ways in which Big Pharma companies can regain public trust and confidence.

Holenz, Jörg, ed. 2016. *Lead Generation: Methods, Strategies, and Case Studies*. 2 vols. Weinheim, Germany: Wiley-VCH.
The two-volume set of essays provides a comprehensive history and review of current technologies in the discovery of lead compounds, a critical step in the process of drug discovery.

Lesburg, Charles A., ed. 2018. *Modern Approaches in Drug Discovery*. Cambridge, MA: Academic Press.
This fairly technical collection of essays provides an excellent overview of some of the major technologies available to researchers in their search for new drugs.

Loughlin, Keven R., and Joyce A. Generali, eds. 2006. *The Guide to Off-Label Prescription Drugs: New Uses for FDA-Approved Prescription Drugs*. New York: Free Press.

At any one time, numerous drugs have been approved by the U.S. Food and Drug Administration (FDA) for use in treating specific medical disorders. In many cases, those drugs may also be useful in treating conditions not specified by the FDA approval process. Such use is known as *off-label use*. This book lists and discusses more than 1,500 drugs that can be administered for off-label uses.

Mazanov, Jason. 2017. *Managing Drugs in Sport*. New York: Routledge.
    The author argues that athletes always have and always will use drugs, both legal and illegal. Yet sporting groups and organizations tend to ignore that reality and do not develop rational policies and practices for dealing with such issues. He suggests some ways this problem can be resolved.

McKinney, Karen Sue. 2020. *Prescription Drugs: Monitoring, Safety, Use and Management Programs*. New York: Nova Science Publishers.
    This book contains chapters on a variety of prescription drug issues, including data on drug use for youth and adults, safe and effective medicinal uses of opioid pain killers, FDA drug regulation programs, and proposed legislation on prescription drug use.

Opinions throughout History: Drug Use & Abuse. 2018. Amenia, NY: Grey House Publishing.
    This book consists of twenty-eight chapters that deal with the history of psychoactive prescription drugs, dating from about 1860 to the present day.

Peppin, John F., et al., eds. 2018. *Prescription Drug Diversion and Pain: History, Policy, and Treatment*. Oxford: Oxford University Press.

The past few decades have seen a vigorous debate over the use of opioids for the treatment of pain, largely because of the possibility of dangerous, addictive side effects. This collection of essays covers all of the important aspects of that debate, from its history to arguments on both sides of the discussion to the current status of the issue.

Quigley, Fran. 2017. *Prescription for the People: An Activist's Guide to Making Medicine Affordable for All.* Ithaca, NY: ILR Press.

The author argues that, over time, health care systems have changed their focus from finding remedies for human health problems to maximizing profits for big pharmaceutical companies. She explores the evidence for that argument, how the change has occurred, and the steps that can be taken to restore the focus of prescription drug use to better care for individuals.

Reference Shelf: Prescription Drug Abuse. 2017. Amenia, NY: Grey House Publishing.

This book deals with topics such as pain and anxiety in America, drugs for young and old, doctors, big pharma, and solutions related to treatment and policy.

Regitz-Zagrosek, Vera, ed. 2012. *Sex and Gender Differences in Pharmacology.* New York: Springer.

The publisher describes this book as the "very first book to deal with sex and gender differences in drug therapy—an increasingly recognized medical need." Chapters discuss topics such as sex and gender differences in clinical medicine; sex differences in drug effects; sex and gender in adverse drug events, addiction, and placebo; considerations of sex and gender differences in preclinical and clinical trials; and sex and gender differences in several specific disease conditions.

Rosenthal, Martha S. 2019. *Drugs: Mind, Body, and Society*. New York: Oxford University Press.

> This textbook provides a good, general, overall introduction to all aspects of drugs, including statistics on drug use; reasons individuals need and use drugs; how drugs are developed; drug laws, past and present; the nervous system and drug effects; detailed discussions of legal and illegal psychoactive drugs; alcohol; and prescription drugs for psychological disorders.

Schauer, Pete, ed. 2018. *Big Pharma and Drug Pricing*. New York: Greenhaven Publishing.

> This book is part of the Greenhaven series *Opposing Viewpoints*. It contains numerous essays on specific aspects of the drug pricing issue, such as covering the cost of drugs in insurance programs, reasons for the high prices of prescription drugs, the role of competition in reducing drug prices, and the government's role in reducing drug prices.

Schepis, Ty S., ed. 2018. *The Prescription Drug Abuse Epidemic: Incidence, Treatment, Prevention, and Policy*. Santa Barbara, CA: Praeger.

> The seventeen essays that make up this book deal with several specific prescription drugs and drug families, such as opioids, stimulants, and benzodiazepines, as well as general problems of prescription drug abuse, such as abuse issues among young adults and older adults, opioids in emergency settings, and regulation of opioid use in the United States.

Seeman, Mary V. 2010. "Women's Issues in Clinical Trials." In Hertzman, Marc, and Lawrence Adler, eds. *Clinical Trials in Psychopharmacology: A Better Brain*, 2nd ed., Chapter 5. https://doi.org/10.1002/9780470749180.ch5.

> The author provides a broad review of the problems of excluding women from clinical trials, including sections on the history of the problem, perceived advantages in excluding women, changing perspectives on the issue,

the effects of drugs in lactating women, and ethical issues involving risk-benefit analyses.

Temple, Norman J., and Andrew Thompson, eds. 2018. *Excessive Medical Spending: Facing the Challenge*. Boca Raton, FL: CRC Press.

The pricing of prescription drugs reflects several steps in the manufacturer-to-consumer process. The essays in this book discuss issues such as the nuts and bolts of medical research, conflict of interest in research, the process of drug approval and drug regulation, how doctor-prescribing habits are influenced by corporate policies and practices, and ways that the currently overpriced system of prescription drugs can be improved.

Tone, Andrea, and Elizabeth Siegel Watkins, eds. 2007. *Medicating Modern America: Prescription Drugs in History*. New York: New York University Press.

The four essays that make up this book deal with the history of antibiotics, mood stabilizers, hormone replacement drugs, and oral contraceptives.

Articles

Abd-Elsayed, Alaa, et al. 2020. "Prescription Drugs and the US Workforce: Results from a National Safety Council Survey." *Pain Physician*. 23(1): 1–16.

The authors report on a survey of 501 interviews with employers of more than 50 employees as to their perceptions about the significance of prescription drug abuse among their workers. The researchers found that 67 percent of employers had some type and/or level of concern about this problem within their own business.

Adams, Crystal, et al. 2019. "Healthworlds, Cultural Health Toolkits, and Choice: How Acculturation Affects Patients' Views of Prescription Drugs and Prescription Drug

Advertising." *Qualitative Health Research*. 29(10): 1419–1432. doi: 10.1177/1049732319827282.

The authors explore differences in the way minority populations learn about and develop opinions about prescription drugs. They find that those differences have real-world impact on the medication decisions that minority versus whites make.

Ahamed, Akram, et al. 2020. "Analysis of Unregulated Sale of Lifesaving Prescription Drugs Online in the United States," *JAMA Internal Medicine*. 180(4): 607–609. doi:10.1001/jamainternmed.2019.7514.

Many individuals who need life-saving drugs are unable to afford the cost of purchasing those drugs through conventional retail outlets. They turn, instead, to online sources for such drugs. This study explored the relative cost of three drugs—insulin, albuterol, and epinephrine—from both online and conventional sources. They found albuterol inhaler to be about $18 less expensive through retail sources than online, but insulin products $372.30 and $123.19 less expensive online (two forms) than from retail sources.

Anagnostiadis, Eleni, and Sangeeta V. Chatterjee. 2018. "The Dangers of Buying Prescription Drugs from Rogue Wholesale Distributors." *Journal of Medical Regulation*. 104(1): 13–16. https://doi.org/10.30770/2572-1852-104.1.13.

Rogue wholesale drug companies advertise their products to physicians and pharmacies at greatly reduced prices. Those drugs may, however, be dangerous to use. They may not have been approved by the FDA, may not consist of the chemical makeup expected of the drug, may contain harmful ingredients, or may have other defects that make them unsafe and/or ineffective. This article reviews this issue in some detail, with recommendations for ways in which the problem can be controlled.

Aschenbrenner, Diane S. 2019. "FDA Warns of Hidden Prescription Drugs in Dietary Supplements." *The American Journal of Nursing*. 119(5): 22–23. https://journals.lww.com/ajnonline/Fulltext/2019/05000/FDA_Warns_of_Hidden_Prescription_Drugs_in_Dietary.21.aspx.

The author reviews and comments on a recent FDA report noting that some over-the-counter dietary supplements may include in their composition prescription drugs with unlisted additives.

Caplan, Arthur L. 2019. "Obtaining Prescription Drugs in America: It's No Bargain." *Journal of Clinical Investigation*. 129(11): 4558–4559.

The author explains his opinion that "just about everything related to health care in America costs too much."

Carlson, Robert G., et al. 2016. "Predictors of Transition to Heroin Use among Initially Non-Opioid Dependent Illicit Pharmaceutical Opioid Users: A Natural History Study." *Drug and Alcohol Dependence*. 160: 127–134. doi: 10.1016/j.drugalcdep.2015.12.026.

One of the most important drug abuse problems identified in recent years is the rise in heroin addiction rates, often attributed to increasing difficulties in obtaining access to legal prescription drugs. This article explores the relationships between these two trends.

Carr, Teresa. 2017. "Too Many Meds? America's Love Affair with Prescription Medication." *Consumer Reports*. 82(9): 24–39. https://www.consumerreports.org/prescription-drugs/too-many-meds-americas-love-affair-with-prescription-medication/#nation.

The author notes the rapid rise in the sale and consumption of prescription drugs in the United States and points out a number of health and economic problems that have risen as a result of this over-prescription and overuse of such drugs.

Cherubini, Antonio, et al. 2010. "Fighting against Age Discrimination in Clinical Trials." *Journal of the American Geriatric Society.* 58(9): 1791–1796. doi: 10.1111/j.1532-5415.2010.03032.x.

> This article is a report on a meeting held by the European Union of Geriatric Medicine Society, the American Geriatrics Society, FDA, and the European Medicine Agency concerning the practice of excluding older subjects in the clinical trials of new drugs.

Corroon, Jamie, Laurie Mischley, and Michelle Sexton. 2017. "Cannabis as a Substitute for Prescription Drugs—A Cross-Sectional Study." *Journal of Pain Research.* 10: 989–998. doi: 10.2147/JPR.S134330.

> The authors pursue growing evidence that many individuals are switching from prescription (usually opioid) drugs to cannabis as a way of dealing with pain, anxiety, and/or depression. They find new evidence for such a trend.

Daniel, Hilary. 2016. "Stemming the Escalating Cost of Prescription Drugs: A Position Paper of the American College of Physicians." *Annals of Internal Medicine.* 165(1): 50–51. https://doi.org/10.7326/M15-2768.

> This paper is a position statement by the American College of Physicians with regard to the high cost of prescription drugs and the factors that have led to this issue.

DeFrank, Jessica T., et al. 2020. "Direct-to-Consumer Advertising of Prescription Drugs and the Patient–Prescriber Encounter: A Systematic Review." *Health Communications.* 35(6):739–746. doi:10.1080/10410236.2019.1584781.

> This publication is a review of articles in the literature dealing with the practice of direct-to-consumer prescription drug sales, with articles from both the prescriber's and the patient's standpoint about the practice.

Egan, Kathleen L., et al. 2019. "Disposal of Prescription Drugs by Parents of Middle and High School Students." *Journal of Child & Adolescent Substance Abuse.* 28(2): 92–98.

The vast majority of young adults who develop a dependence on or an addiction to drugs begin with exposure to licit prescription drugs. In most cases, they obtain those drugs from friends and family. The purpose of this study was to determine the methods used by parents to dispose of unused prescription medications. Researchers found that less than 20 percent of parents disposed of such drugs by any method at all.

Feldman, William B., et al. 2020. "Estimation of Medicare Part D Spending on Insulin for Patients with Diabetes Using Negotiated Prices and a Defined Formulary." *JAMA Internal Medicine.* 180(4): 597–601. doi:10.1001/jamainternmed.2019.7018.

Government agencies use different systems for negotiating and paying the price of prescription drugs that they provide their populations of consumers. This study found that having Medicare use the system currently practiced by the Veterans Administration would save them $4.4 billion annually on the purchase of insulin alone from their current expenditure of $7.8 billion, a saving of more than 56 percent.

Gassman, Audrey L., Christine P. Nguyen, and Hylton V. Joffe. 2017. "FDA Regulation of Prescription Drugs." *New England Journal of Medicine.* 376(7): 674–682. doi:10.1056/NEJMra1602972.

This article provides a simple, complete introduction to the process by which FDA approves new prescription drugs.

Gluud, Lise Lotte. 2006. "Bias in Clinical Intervention Research." *American Journal of Epidemiology.* 163(6): 493–501. https://doi.org/10.1093/aje/kwj069.

The author explains why biases in clinical testing may cause significant false results for the interpretation of results and how such problems can be avoided.

Goldstein, Daniel A., and Michal Sarfatya. 2016. "Cancer Drug Pricing and Reimbursement: Lessons for the United States from around the World." *Oncologist*. 21(8): 907–909. doi:10.1634/theoncologist.2016-0106.

Systems for the pricing of cancer drugs around the world provide a good review of the reason that prescription drug prices are so much higher in the United States than they are in most other countries worldwide. This article reviews those data for a variety of nations.

Hales, Craig M., et al. 2018. "Trends in Prescription Medication Use among Children and Adolescents—United States, 1999–2014." *JAMA*. 319(19): 2009–2020. doi:10.1001/jama.2018.5690.

This article reports on a survey of prescription drugs used by children and adolescents during the period from 1999 to 2014. Researchers found a modest decrease in prescription drugs used for antibiotics, antihistamines, and upper respiratory combination medications and a modest increase in drugs used for asthma medications, attention deficit hyperactivity disorder medications, proton pump inhibitors, and contraceptives.

Harbut, Rachel F., and Danielle Hahn Chaet. 2019. "AMA Code of Medical Ethics' Opinions Related to Prescription Drugs." *AMA Journal of Ethics*. 21(8): E642–E644. https://journalofethics.ama-assn.org/sites/journalofethics.ama-assn.org/files/2019-07/code1-1908.pdf.

The American Medical Association maintains a Code of Ethics that deals with a host of issues with which physicians might become involved. This article summarizes some of the opinions that the society has issued on problems relating to prescription drugs, with links to detailed discussions of each such opinion.

Hilal, Maha, et al. 2017. "Chemistry, Pharmacology and Toxicology of New Designer Drugs—A Comprehensive Review." *Sohag Medical Journal.* 21(1): 205–214. doi:10.21608/smj.2017.40735.
This article provides a good general introduction to the nature, history, and current status of designer drugs.

Huestis, M. A., and R. F. Tyndale. 2017. "Designer Drugs 2.0." *Clinical Pharmacology & Therapeutics.* 101(2): 152–157.
This article is an introduction to a special issue of the journal dealing with the current status of research on designer drugs. It outlines the development of new drugs and the repurposing of traditional drugs for new uses.

Hughes, J. P., et al. 2011. "Principles of Early Drug Discovery." *British Journal of Pharmacology.* 162(6): 1239–1249. doi:10.1111/j.1476-5381.2010.01127.x.
This excellent article provides a clear and comprehensive review of the steps that occur in the process of early drug discovery, from the earliest steps of basic research to the selection of a candidate molecule.

Hwang, Thomas J., Aaron S. Kesselheim, and Ameet Sarpatwari. 2017. "Value-Based Pricing and State Reform of Prescription Drug Costs." *JAMA.* 318(7): 609–610. doi:10.1001/jama.2017.8255.
One of the methods proposed for dealing with rising drug prices is value-based pricing, a system by which the price of a prescription drug is based on the perceived value of the drug to the user, not on some other criterion, such as profit to the company. This article discusses the concept of value-based pricing and its first state implementation (New York state) in 2017.

Jarow, Jonathan P., et al. 2017. "Overview of FDA's Expanded Access Program for Investigational Drugs." *Therapeutic Innovation and Regulatory Science.* 51(2): 177–179. doi:10.1177/2168479017694850.

In 1987, the FDA modified its requirements for the approval of a new candidate drug in order to accommodate individuals with serious diseases and/or disorders for whom no alternative therapies were currently available. This article reviews the history and current status of that program. The program is commonly referred to as "compassionate use" of prescription drugs.

Kacinko, Sherri L., and Donna M. Papsun. 2019. "The Evolving Landscape of Designer Drugs." *Methods in Molecular Biology.* 1872: 129–135.

The authors provide an excellent general introduction to the history of designer drugs, a discussion of their action in the body, and a review of current developments in the field.

Langjahr, Allen. 2020. "Prescription Drugs and Pricing Transparency." *US Pharmacist.* 45(1): 34–36. https://www.uspharma cist.com/article/prescription-drugs-and-pricing-transparency.

In November 2019, President Donald Trump issued a pair of new rules that would increase the transparency of information about drug costs: the Hospital Price Transparency Rule and the Transparency in Coverage Rule. This article describes these rules and their relevance for drug purchasing by the general public.

Li, Meng, and Mark Bounthavong. 2020. "Medicare Beneficiaries, Especially Unsubsidized Minorities, Struggle to Pay for Prescription Drugs: Results from the Medicare Current Beneficiary Survey." *Journal of General Internal Medicine.* 35(4): 1334–1336. https://doi.org/10.1007/s11606-019-05204-2.

Researchers have known for some time that Medicare Part D benefits are often inadequate for the payment of drug costs among a significant portion of the American public, especially minorities who do not have access to this program. This article provides the most recent data indicating that this is still a major problem in the American health care system.

Luethi, Dino, and Matthias E. Liechti. 2020. "Designer Drugs: Mechanism of Action and Adverse Effects." *Archives of Toxicology*. 94(4): 1085–1133. https://doi.org/10.1007/s00 204-020-02693-7.
This superb article is a good introduction to the basics of designer drugs along with a more detailed and technical discussion of their modes of action in the human body.

Mello, Michelle M. 2018. "What Makes Ensuring Access to Affordable Prescription Drugs the Hardest Problem in Health Policy?" *Minnesota Law Review*. 102(6): 2273–2305. https://law.stanford.edu/wp-content/uploads/2018/07/Mello_ MLR.pdf.
The author draws on her own experience of trying to find less expensive prescription drugs for her food allergic child. She concludes that, while prescription drug costs are part of an overall problem with health care costs in the United States, the issue "is also plagued by distinctive moral, market, and political problems . . . especially the lack of transparency."

Mello, Michelle M. 2020. "Barriers to Ensuring Access to Affordable Prescription Drugs." *Annual Review of Pharmacology and Toxicology*. 60(1): 275–289. https://doi.org/10.1146/ annurev-pharmtox-010919-023518.
The author notes that the high cost of prescription drugs has been a difficult problem in the United States for many years. She suggests there are moral, market, and political factors responsible for the inertia in solving this issue. She discusses each type of issue here.

Morgan, Steven G., et al. 2018. "An Analysis of Expenditures on Primary Care Prescription Drugs in the United States versus Ten Comparable Countries." *Health Policy.* 122(9): 1012–1017. https://doi.org/10.1016/j.healthpol.2018.07.005.

The authors explored price differences between prescription drugs in the United States and those in ten "comparable countries." Drugs used in the study were those for hypertension treatments, pain medications, lipid-lowing medicines, non-insulin diabetes treatments, gastrointestinal preparations, and treatments for depression. They found that Americans spend 203 percent more for comparable prescription drugs in the United States than in the comparison countries. By reducing this differential, Americans could save more than $21 billion annually on drug costs.

Mukherjee, Samrat Kumar, et al. 2019. "Role of Social Media Promotion of Prescription Drugs on Patient Belief—System and Behaviour." *International Journal of e-Collaboration.* 15(2): 23–43.

The authors suggest that there is little research on the ways in which social media information on prescription drugs affects the attitudes and practices of patients with regard to prescription drug use. They conclude that such sources of information can provide valuable and useful information for patients, but problems may arise in the reliance on social media for such information.

Nelson, Roxanne. 2015. "The Excessive Waste of Prescription Drugs." *The American Journal of Nursing.* 115(6): 19–20. doi:10.1097/01.NAJ.0000466308.08390.7b.

The author discusses one of the less commonly reviewed problems of prescription drugs, namely, the number of such drugs that are prescribed but never used. She outlines some ways of dealing with this problem.

Neumann, Peter J., and Joshua T. Cohen. 2015. "Measuring the Value of Prescription Drugs." *New England Journal of Medicine.* 373(27): 2595–2597. doi:10.1056/NEJMp1512009.

The authors describe a new method for assessing the value of prescription drugs of growing interest in the medical profession. The method is based on the use of a variety of factors, including quality of clinical data supporting the therapy's use, the magnitude of its treatment effects, the likelihood of severe adverse events, and the product's costs, ancillary benefits, cost effectiveness, and effects on the health system budget.

Oluwoye, Oladunni A., Ashley L. Merianos, and Laura A. Nabors. 2017. "Nonmedical Use of Prescription Drugs and Peer Norms among Adolescents by Race/Ethnicity." *Journal of Substance Use*. 22(2): 199–205.

This article summarizes data on the nonmedical use of prescription drugs among various categories of adolescents. The data show that each group responds to this practice in a somewhat different ways from other groups.

Persaud, Navindra, et al. 2019. "Effect on Treatment Adherence of Distributing Essential Medicines at No Charge: The CLEAN Meds Randomized Clinical Trial." *JAMA Internal Medicine*. 180(1): 27–34. doi:10.1001/jamainternmed.2019.4472.

One serious problem with the use of prescription drugs is that a significant number of individuals who are prescribed such products do not take them as intended. The expense of the drug is often a major factor in this pattern. This study examines the behavior of patients who are prescribed a drug at no cost to them. It finds that adherence to the drug schedule is higher when the drugs are free.

"Pharaohs and the First Prescriptions." 2007. *Pharmaceutical Journal*. 279(7483): 735–737. https://www.pharmaceutical-journal.com/news-and-analysis/features/pharaohs-and-the-first-prescriptions/10005731.article.

This article reviews some of the earliest prescriptions known, produced as far back as about 1800 BCE.

Pharmacy in History. Quarterly Journal. ISSN: 0031-7047 (print); 2329-5031 (online). https://aihp.org/pharmacy-in-history-journal/.

The American Institute of the History of Pharmacy publishes this peer-reviewed journal, containing articles on the history of pharmacy and pharmaceuticals. Some interesting articles about the history of prescription drugs are to be found in issues of the journal.

Rajkumar, Vincent S. 2020. "The High Cost of Prescription Drugs: Causes and Solutions." *Blood Cancer Journal.* 10(71). https://doi.org/10.1038/s41408-020-0338-x.

The author provides a relatively simple and comprehensive review of the factors that lead to the high cost of prescription drugs and steps that can be taken to deal with that problem.

Reiff, Mark R. 2019. "The Just Price, Exploitation, and Prescription Drugs: Why Free Marketeers Should Object to Profiteering by the Pharmaceutical Industry." *Review of Social Economy.* 77(2): 108–142.

The author notes that free-market economics generally have no problem with prescription drug costs since they simply reflect market forces relating to the topic. He points out, however, that such is not the case and that prescription drug prices ought to be an issue of considerable importance to this group of professionals.

Sachs, Rachel E., and Nicholas Bagley. 2020. "Importing Prescription Drugs from Canada—Legal and Practical Problems with the Trump Administration's Proposal." *New England Journal of Medicine.* 382(19): 1777–1779.

In 2020, President Donald Trump proposed a plan by which Americans would be able to purchase prescription drugs, supposedly at reduced prices, from Canadian sources. The authors of this article explain why such a plan is unlikely to be successful and may also be illegal.

Schifano, Fabrizio, et al. 2018. "Abuse of Prescription Drugs in the Context of Novel Psychoactive Substances (NPS): A Systematic Review." *Brain Sciences*. 8(4): 73. doi:10.3390/brainsci8040073.

> This excellent paper provides a review of the current status of novel psychoactive substances (NPS). It focuses on some of the most popular drugs in that category currently available, with detailed discussions of the harms they may pose to users. The authors conclude that NPSs are "a challenge for psychiatry, public health and drug-control policies."

Seligman, Paul J., et al. 2019. "Managing the Risks of Medicines: An Examination of FDA's Application of Criteria for Requiring a REMS." *Therapeutic Innovation & Regulatory Science*. 53(4): 542–548. https://doi.org/10.1177/2168479018791560.

> The FDA published a "draft guidance for industry" document in 2016 outlining the rationale for issuing risk evaluation and mitigation strategies (REMS) for certain specific drugs. This article reviews the FDA's actions on 113 new products for which REMS was being considered. The FDA eventually selected only five of those drugs for REMS action. The article analyzes and discusses the criteria on which these decisions were made.

Serdarevic, Mirsada, et al. 2020. "If Kids Ruled the World, How Would They Stop the Non-Medical Use of Prescription Drugs?" *Journal of Health Research*. Emerald Insight. https://doi.org/10.1108/JHR-02-2019-0031.

> As part of the National Monitoring of Adolescent Prescription Stimulants Study, a selection of young adults were asked how they would act to reduce the illegal use of prescription drugs. The respondents suggested providing more and better education about prescription drugs and their negative effects at schools, by parents and health professionals and through the media. They also

recommended more stringent laws that restricted use and providing education about negative consequences of use.

Smirnova, Michelle, and Jennifer Gatewood Owens. 2019. "The New Mothers' Little Helpers: Medicalization, Victimization, and Criminalization of Motherhood via Prescription Drugs." *Deviant Behavior*. 40(8): 957–970. https://doi.org/10.1080/01639625.2018.1449433.

> In this study of forty incarcerated women, nearly three quarters were prescribed prescription drugs to recover from cesarean deliveries. The majority of those women eventually concluded that the use of those drugs aided them in the care of their newborn children.

Thomas, Sherine E., et al. 2017. "Structural Biology and the Design of New Therapeutics: From HIV and Cancer to Mycobacterial Infections." *Journal of Molecular Biology*. 429: 2677–2693. https://doi.org/10.1016/j.jmb.2017.06.014.

> This paper outlines the process of target identification, the discovery of characteristic structural features of a substance at which a candidate drug will be able to bind and, therefore, exert an effect.

Thompson, R. Campbell. 1929. "Assyrian Medical Prescriptions for Diseases of the Stomach." *Revue d'assyriologie et d'archéologie Orientale*. 26(2): 47–92.

> The author reprints translations of many prescriptions discovered for the treatment of stomach disorders by Assyrian healers.

Van der Gronde, Toon, Carin A. Uyl-de Groot, and Toine Pieters. 2017. "Addressing the Challenge of High-Priced Prescription Drugs in the Era of Precision Medicine: A Systematic Review of Drug Life Cycles, Therapeutic Drug Markets and Regulatory Frameworks." *PLOS One*. E 12(8): e0182613. https://doi.org/10.1371/journal.pone.0182613.

Countries around the world have designed a variety of methods for dealing with the high cost of health care, in general, and of prescription drugs, in particular. Some of the methods explored in this article are patent reform legislation, reference pricing, outcome-based pricing, and incentivizing physicians and pharmacists to prescribe low-cost drugs.

Wechsler, Jill. 2017. "Measuring the Value of Prescription Drugs." *Pharmaceutical Executive.* 37(5): 10. http://www.phar mexec.com/measuring-value-prescription-drugs.

One approach to resolving the problem of prescription drug costs is a system known as "measuring the value" of prescription drugs. This system takes into account several factors involving the relative therapeutic and economic value of a drug, compared to other products of the same type.

Yantsides, Konstantina E., Migdalia R. Tracy, and Margie Skeer. 2017. "Non-Medical Use of Prescription Drugs and Its Association with Heroin Use among High School Students." *Journal of Substance Use.* 22(1): 102–107.

The authors note that the relationship between non-medical use of prescription drugs and heroin use is well studied for adults but poorly understood for adolescents. They report on the data they collected on this question and note that a correlation between the two practices exists in varying degrees for males, those carrying a weapon in the past thirty days, and sexually active individuals, dating violence victimization, and reporting other drug use.

Zafar, S. Yousuf, and Amy P. Abernethy. 2013. "Financial Toxicity, Part I: A New Name for a Growing Problem." *Oncology.* 27(2): 80–149. https://www.ncbi.nlm.nih.gov/pmc/articles/ PMC4523887/.

Financial toxicity is a relatively new term that refers to possible effects that may result from one's inability to pay one's necessary medical costs. Those effects may include both economic issues (debt and bankruptcy) and physical and mental health issues (depression and stress). This is the first of two articles on the topic, the second being S. Yousuf Zafar and Amy P. Abernethy. 2013. "Financial Toxicity, Part II: How Can We Help with the Burden of Treatment-Related Costs?" *Oncology.* 27(4): 253–254, 256. https://www.cancernetwork.com/view/financial-toxicity-part-ii-how-can-we-help-burden-treatment-related-costs.

Ziavrou, Kalliroi. 2018. "New Psychoactive Substances: Challenges for Law Enforcement Agencies and the Law." George C. Marshall European Center for Security Studies. https://www.marshallcenter.org/en/publications/occasional-papers/new-psychoactive-substances-challenges-law-enforcement-agencies-and-law.

The author explores legal issues associated with the invention, development, distribution, use, and dangers posed by designed drugs (new psychoactive substances).

Reports

Augustine, Norman R., Guru Madhavan, and Sharyl J. Nass, eds. 2018. *Making Medicines Affordable: A National Imperative.* Washington, D.C.: The National Academies Press. https://doi.org/10.17226/24946.

This report is one of the most detailed and most extensive of recent efforts to understand the issues of prescription drug costs and methods for making such drugs more readily affordable for the general public. The four major sections are The Affordability Conundrum, Complexity in Action, Factors Affecting Affordability, and Strategies to Improve Affordability and Availability.

Bonnie, Richard J., Morgan A. Ford, and Jonathan Phillips, eds. 2017. *Pain Management and the Opioid Epidemic: Balancing Societal and Individual Benefits and Risks of Prescription Opioid Use.* Washington, D.C.: The National Academies Press.
This report reviews the current status of the prescription drug/opioid drug crisis, the factors responsible for its development, and steps that can be taken to reduce the problem in the future.

Cauchi, Richard. 2018. State Remedies for Costly Prescription Drugs. National Conference of State Legislatures. https://www.ncsl.org/research/health/state-remedies-for-costly-prescription-drugs.aspx.
This report reviews some of the methods that state legislatures have adopted for dealing with the problem of prescription drug abuse, including the prohibition of "gag clauses," which prevent pharmacists from informing customers about lower-price generic drugs, promoting drug price transparency, prohibiting drug price gouging, and promoting "free speech" in medicine.

Center for Sustainable Health. 2014. Spending Data Brief: A 10-Year Projection of the Prescription Drug Share of National Health Expenditures, Including Nonretail. Altarum Institute. https://altarum.org/sites/default/files/uploaded-publication-files/Non-Retail%20Rx%20Forecast%20Data%20Brief%2010-14-14.pdf.
Most discussions of prescription drug costs focus primarily on retail prices, the price paid for a drug distributed through pharmacies, food stores, mail order companies, department stores, and other mass providers. They often do not include data from nonretail sources, such as physicians' offices and hospitals. This study is one of an increasing number that attempt to include estimates of nonretail drug costs as well as retail drug costs.

CMS Drug Spending. 2019. Centers for Medicare and Medicaid Services. https://www.cms.gov/Research-Statistics-Data-and-Systems/Statistics-Trends-and-Reports/Informa tion-on-Prescription-Drugs.

This web page explains and provides links to data collections on drugs used in Part B, Part D, and Medicaid programs, including average spending per dosage unit and change in average spending per dosage unit over time, manufacturer-level drug spending information, and consumer-friendly descriptions of the drug uses and clinical indications.

College Prescription Drug Study. 2018. The Ohio State University. https://www.campusdrugprevention.gov/sites/default/files/2018%20College%20Prescription%20Drug%20Study .pdf.

This study reviewed prescription drug use and abuse among 19,539 students at 26 institutions of higher learning in the United States. It asked about topics such as frequency of use, access to prescription drugs, reasons for use, consequences of use, education and resources, and prescribed medication behaviors.

Drug Utilization Review Annual Report. 2018 [Annual]. Medicaid.gov. https://www.medicaid.gov/medicaid/prescription-drugs/drug-utilization-review/drug-utilization-review-annual-report/index.html.

States are required by federal law to report data on practitioner prescribing habits, drug costs, and program operation to Medicaid. This long and detailed report summarizes the results of such a survey for all states and as federal averages. The report contains 137 figures and 193 tables of data.

Kirzinger, Ashley, et al. 2019. KFF Health Tracking Poll—February 2019: Prescription Drugs. Kaiser Family Foundation.

https://www.kff.org/health-costs/poll-finding/kff-health-tracking-poll-february-2019-prescription-drugs/.

This poll tracks public opinion on a variety of questions relating to prescription drugs, such as their importance in individuals' lives, their cost, trust in pharmaceutical companies, and views on governmental and political suggestions for dealing with prescription drug costs and availability.

Kleinrock, Michael, and Elyse Muñoz. 2020. Global Medicine Spending and Usage Trends: Outlook to 2024. IQVIA Institute. https://www.iqvia.com/-/media/iqvia/pdfs/institute-reports/global-medicine-spending-and-usage-trends.pdf.

IQVIA Institute publishes an annual review of the global status of medications. This report is the 2020 version of that series.

Misuse of Prescription Drugs Research Report. 2020. National Institute on Drug Abuse, National Institutes of Health, U.S. Department of Health and Human Services. https://www.drugabuse.gov/download/37630/misuse-prescription-drugs-research-report.pdf.

This report discusses the current status of prescription drug abuse in the United States, with chapters on the scope of the problem, the use of prescription drugs in combination with other medicines, the types of drugs most commonly misused, the use of prescription drugs during pregnancy, how prescription drug abuse can be prevented, and how prescription drug abuse can be treated.

Mossialos, Elias, et al. 2016. 2015 International Profiles of Health Care Systems. The Commonwealth Fund. https://www.commonwealthfund.org/sites/default/files/documents/___media_files_publications_fund_report_2016_jan_1857_mossialos_intl_profiles_2015_v7.pdf.

The United States has been called "an outlier" in terms of prescription drug pricing because its system for setting prices is so different from that of most other countries in the world. This report reviews the systems for prescription drug pricing and related topics in seventeen nations: Australia, Canada, China, Denmark, England, France, Germany, India, Israel, Italy, Japan, The Netherlands, New Zealand, Norway, Singapore, Sweden, Switzerland, as well as the United States.

National Academies of Sciences, Engineering, and Medicine. 2020. *Framing Opioid Prescribing Guidelines for Acute Pain: Developing the Evidence.* Washington, D.C.: The National Academies Press. https://doi.org/10.17226/25555.

An important element in the prescription drug abuse epidemic has been the fact that health care workers routinely overprescribe the amount of pain killers a person may need. These "leftover" pills then end up in a medicine cabinet or another location where they can be accessed by individuals with an opioid use problem. This report attempts to develop guidelines for the prescribing of opioid medicines to reduce this problem.

Office of the Assistant Secretary for Planning and Evaluation. 2016. Prescription Drugs: Innovation, Spending, and Patient Access. U.S. Department of Health and Human Services. https://aspe.hhs.gov/system/files/pdf/262751/DrugPricingR TC2016.pdf.

This report to the U.S. Congress provides detailed information about the type, cost, trends, uses, and other data concerning new drug development and implementation in Medicare Part B, Medicare Part D, Medicaid, and the Veterans Health Administration.

The Prescription Drug Landscape, Explored. 2019. The Pew Charitable Trusts. https://www.pewtrusts.org/-/media/ assets/2019/03/the_prescription_drug_landscape-explored. pdf.

This report focuses on the changing costs of prescription drugs between 2012 and 2016, with substantial detail on the ways in which those costs are incurred by patients, drug companies, and other entities in society.

Rosenberg, Alex. 2019. Prescription Drugs: Path to Patient. Legislative Reference Bureau. https://docs.legis.wisconsin.gov/misc/lrb/wisconsin_policy_project/wisconsin_policy_project_2_3.pdf.
This report for the State of Wisconsin legislature provides a superb and easily understood overview of the economics involved in the production, distribution, and use of prescription drugs.

2019 National Drug Threat Assessment. 2019. Drug Enforcement Administration. https://www.dea.gov/sites/default/files/2020-01/2019-NDTA-final-01-14-2020_Low_Web-DIR-007-20_2019.pdf.
This document reports on the current status of the most commonly misused prescription drugs, including fentanyl, heroin, cocaine, and new psychoactive substances, as well as important general issues, such as transnational criminal organizations, tribal threats, and illicit financing.

Ways and Means Committee Staff. 2019. A Painful Pill to Swallow: U.S. vs. International Prescription Drug Prices. Committee on Ways and Means, U.S. House of Representatives. https://waysandmeans.house.gov/sites/democrats.waysandmeans.house.gov/files/documents/U.S.%20vs.%20International%20Prescription%20Drug%20Prices_0.pdf.
This report compares the prices of prescription drugs in the United States with those of ten foreign countries and one Canadian province: United Kingdom, Japan, Australia, Portugal, France, the Netherlands, Germany, Denmark, Sweden, Switzerland, and Ontario. It finds that the average price of prescription drugs in the United

States is about four times that for similar drugs in the comparison nation and that Americans could save about $49 billion annually if drug prices in the United States were comparable to those in the comparison nations and province.

Internet

The American Cancer Society Medical and Editorial Content Team. 2017. "Prescription Drugs to Help You Quit Tobacco." American Cancer Society. https://www.cancer.org/healthy/stay-away-from-tobacco/guide-quitting-smoking/prescription-drugs-to-help-you-quit-smoking.html#written_by.

Individuals who are attempting to quit smoking may find certain prescription drugs helpful in this effort. This article discusses the positive and negative aspects of a handful of such drugs in such a program.

Armstrong, John, and Colleen Beckere. 2019. "Value-Based Pricing to Address Drug Costs." National Conference of State Legislatures. https://www.ncsl.org/research/health/value-based-pricing-to-address-drug-costs.aspx.

States have been exploring methods for reducing the rapidly rising cost of prescription drugs by pursuing alternative payment models, that is, the setting of prices for prescription drugs using a method other than the traditional method of allowing pharmaceutical companies to set those prices using their own criteria. One of the most popular of these methods is called *value-based pricing*. That system is explained here, and its progress through various state legislatures is reviewed.

Booth, Bruce. 2016. "Innovators vs. Exploiters: Drug Pricing and the Future of Pharma." *Forbes.* https://www.forbes.com/sites/brucebooth/2016/08/29/innovators-vs-exploiters-drug-pricing-and-the-future-of-pharma.

The author explores the role played by two types of drug manufacturers—those who actually discover new drugs, the innovators, and those who make use of those discoveries to produce generic equivalents, the exploiters—in the current rise in drug prices in the United States.

Bowsher, Karla. "4 Grocery Store Chains That Offer Free Prescription Drugs." 2019. Yahoo Finance. https://finance.yahoo.com/news/8-grocery-store-chains-offer-231520981.html.
Many consumers may not be aware of the fact that some types of prescription drugs can be obtained at no cost from certain commercial outlets. This article explains how that it is possible and some sources of free prescription drugs.

"A Brief History of the Center for Drug Evaluation and Research." 2018. U.S. Food and Drug Administration. https://www.fda.gov/about-fda/virtual-exhibits-fda-history/brief-history-center-drug-evaluation-and-research.
The Center for Drug Evaluation and Research is the entity within the FDA responsible for reviewing and acting on data and other information provided by pharmaceutical companies in their research for possible candidate molecules for new drugs.

Coppock, Kristen. 2019. "Policy Makers Seek Answers for High Costs of Prescription Drugs." *Pharmacy Times*. https://www.pharmacytimes.com/news/policy-makers-seek-answers-for-high-costs-of-prescription-drugs.
This article is a summary of hearings held by the House Committee on Energy & Commerce on the high cost of prescription drugs. A committee summary of the meetings can be found at https://www.congress.gov/116/meeting/house/109436/documents/HHRG-116-IF14-20190509-SD002.pdf, and a video of a portion of the session can be found at https://energycommerce.house.gov/committee-activity/hearings/hearing-on-lowering-prescription-drug-prices-deconstructing-the-drug.

"DEA National Takeback." 2020. Drug Enforcement Administration. https://takebackday.dea.gov/.

    The DEA regularly sponsors a national Takeback Day, during which individuals can legally and safely dispose of unused prescription medications. This website provides details about that program.

Dolan, Rachel. 2019. "Understanding the Medicaid Prescription Drug Rebate Program." Kaiser Family Foundation. https://www.kff.org/medicaid/issue-brief/understanding-the-medicaid-prescription-drug-rebate-program/.

    The Medicaid Prescription Drug Rebate Program is a program by which drug companies agree to reduce the cost of a prescription drug they charge to states in return for the federal government's listing the drug as an approved Medicaid drug. This article discusses that program in detail and provides examples of the ways in which it works.

"Drug Companies as Taxpayer Funding Boosts Bottom Lines; Billions of Dollars Distributed to Shareholders, Executives." 2020. Accountable.us. https://www.accountable.us/news/another-big-quarter-for-drug-companies-as-taxpayer-funding-boosts-bottom-lines-billions-of-dollars-distributed-to-shareholders-executives/.

    This brief article summarizes financial reports from nine major pharmaceutical companies, including special grants they received for research on the COVID-19 pandemic.

"Drug Development." 2020. Science Direct. https://www.sciencedirect.com/topics/nursing-and-health-professions/drug-development.

    This website lists several books, articles, and other resources providing basic information on the process of drug development.

"The Drug Development Process." 2018. U.S. Food and Drug Administration. https://www.fda.gov/patients/learn-about-drug-and-device-approvals/drug-development-process.

This website provides a complete and readable review of the steps that occur in the process of a new drug development.

"Drug Index A to Z." 2020. Drugs.com. https://www.drugs .com/drug_information.html.
An extensive collection of basic information on more than 24,000 prescription and over-the-counter medications.

"Drugs & Medications A–Z." 2020. WebMD. https://www .webmd.com/drugs/2/index.
This website is an excellent resource for reviews of hundreds of drugs and other types of medications, ranging from aspirin to Zavesca.

"Executive Order on Increasing Drug Importation to Lower Prices for American Patients." 2020. The White House. https:// www.govinfo.gov/content/pkg/DCPD-202000540/html/ DCPD-202000540.htm.
In July 2020, President Donald Trump issued an Executive Order announcing a new policy making it easier for Americans to order prescription drugs online from other countries. This website contains the text of that document.

"FDA Update—The FDA's New Drug Approval Process: Development & Premarket Applications." 2018. Drug Development & Delivery. https://drug-dev.com/fda-update-the-fdas-new-drug-approval-process-development-premarket-applications/.
The original FDA system for drug approval and delivery was issued in 2004. This document describes in detail the provisions of that document as well as changes that have been made in the process more recently. The article goes well beyond a simple review of the drug development process to discussing the details involved at every step of that process.

"Featured Prescription Drugs Resources." 2020. KFF. https:// www.kff.org/tag/prescription-drugs/.

The Kaiser Family Foundation is one of the most trusted organizations for information on a host of health care issues. This web page lists many articles on the topic of prescription drugs that have recently appeared on their website.

"Frequently Asked Questions about Prescription Drug Pricing and Policy." 2018. Congressional Research Service. https://crsreports.congress.gov/product/pdf/R/R44832.

This report provides a good general summary of the basic facts of prescription drug costs in the United States, including recent data, explanations for data trends, governmental role in the prescription drug spending issue, and pharmaceutical development and marketing.

Hayes, Tara O'Neill. 2018. "Is an International Price Index the Solution to High Drug Prices?" American Action Forum. https://www.americanactionforum.org/insight/is-an-international-price-index-the-solution-to-high-drug-prices/.

Under current programs, Medicare pays for the cost of prescription drugs based on the average price of those drugs in the private marketplace. Another way to determine such prices is called an international price index (IPI), which is based on the average price of drugs paid by other countries in the world that set those prices at a national level. This article reviews proposals by the Trump administration to text an IPI that would be based on the average drug prices in sixteen countries where drugs are priced by federal authorities.

"How to Buy and Use Medicine." 2019. USA.gov. https://www.usa.gov/medicine.

This website provides a very useful, comprehensive overview of questions relating to the purchase and use of prescription drugs. It deals with questions such as what help is available to pay for prescription drugs, whether a person is eligible for help in dealing with prescription drug costs, how one applies for prescription drug cost assistance, pet medication problems, dietary supplements, and complaints about prescription drug–related issues.

"How to Get Prescription Drug Coverage." n.d. Medicare.gov. https://www.medicare.gov/drug-coverage-part-d/how-to-get-prescription-drug-coverage.
This web page is intended for individuals interested in obtaining prescription drug coverage through the Medicare program. It gives the detailed process to go through for that purpose.

"How Will the Rising Cost of Prescription Drugs Affect Medicare?" 2018. Peter G. Peterson Foundation. https://www.pgpf.org/blog/2018/09/how-will-the-rising-cost-of-prescription-drugs-affect-medicare.
This article places the problem of rising drug costs into the more general question as to how these changes are likely to affect the function of Medicare itself. The article provides some excellent data on the issue.

Junod, Suzanne White. 2008. "FDA and Clinical Drug Trials: A Short History." https://www.fda.gov/media/110437/download.
This excellent article provides a good review of the stages through which the FDA drug approval process in use today has evolved over time.

Kamal, Rabah, Cynthis Cox, and Daniel McDermott. 2019. "What Are the Recent and Forecasted Trends in Prescription Drug Spending?" Peterson-KFF Health System Tracker. https://www.healthsystemtracker.org/chart-collection/recent-forecasted-trends-prescription-drug-spending/#item-start.
This excellent article provides an extensive summary of current statistical information on the costs of prescription

drugs, along with some reliable projections for future patterns on this topic.

Kapoor, D., R. B. Vyas, and D. Dadarwal. 2018. "An Overview on Pharmaceutical Supply Chain: A Next Step towards Good Manufacturing Practice." *Drug Designing & Intellectual Properties International Journal.* doi:10.32474/DDIPIJ.2018.01.000107.
   This article provides a good general introduction to the steps involved in a drug supply chain, along with a discussion of steps that can be taken to ensure the integrity of each of those steps in maintaining the safety of a drug product.

Kliff, Sarah. 2018. "The True Story of America's Sky-High Prescription Drug Prices." Vox. https://www.vox.com/science-and-health/2016/11/30/12945756/prescription-drug-prices-explained.
   The method by which prescription drug prices are set in the United States is different from that of most other countries around the world. This article discusses the way in which prescription drug prices are set in Australia, Canada, Great Britain, and other developed countries.

Landsdowne, Laura Elizabeth. 2018. "Target Identification & Validation in Drug Discovery." Technology Networks. https://www.technologynetworks.com/drug-discovery/articles/target-identification-validation-in-drug-discovery-312290.
   A critical aspect in the process of drug discovery in today's world is target identification, the determination of any set of atoms, radicals, molecules, or other species to which a proposed drug must bind in order for it to take effect. This article outlines the main features of the target identification process.

Lin, Judy, and Elizabeth Aguilera. 2020. "Gov. Gavin Newsom to Propose That California Manufacture its Own Generic

Drugs." Cal Matters. https://calmatters.org/health/2020/01/gavin-newsom-to-propose-california-manufacture-state-generic-drugs/.

In 2020, California governor Gavin Newsom proposed the creation of a state-owned and -operated pharmaceutical company for the purpose of producing prescription drugs at lower prices than those available from existing companies. This article provides a review of that proposal and possible outcomes it may or may not produce. Newsom's plan is somewhat similar to a proposal released by Senator Elizabeth Warren in her run for the Democratic nomination for president in 2018. See "Warren, Schakowsky Introduce Bicameral Legislation to Radically Reduce Drug Prices through Public Manufacturing of Prescription Drugs."

Lipari, Rachel N., Matthew Williams, and Struther L. Van Horn. 2017. "Why Do Adults Misuse Prescription Drugs?" Rockville, MD: U.S. Department of Health and Human Services, Substance Abuse and Mental Health Services Administration. https://www.samhsa.gov/data/sites/default/files/report_3210/ShortReport-3210.html.

This article summarizes the findings of the 2015 National Survey on Drug Use and Health regarding the status of prescription drug abuse by adults in the United States.

Lippmann, Elaine. 2017. "Risk Evaluation and Mitigation Strategies (REMS)." U.S. Food and Drug Administration. https://www.fda.gov/media/105565/download.

This slide presentation provides an understandable and comprehensive explanation of the theory and practice of risk evaluation and mitigation strategies. Also see "Risk Evaluation and Mitigation Strategies: REMS."

Llamas, Michelle. 2020. "Misplaced Trust: Why FDA Approval Doesn't Guarantee Drug Safety." DrugWatch. https://www.drugwatch.com/featured/misplaced-trust-fda-approval-concerns/.

This article provides an overview of the procedures by which FDA approves drugs, along with special programs, such as compassionate use of drugs. It then suggests several ways in which this process is less than satisfactory and may actually result in the approval of drugs that are not safe for human consumption.

Marwah, Upasana, Dana Huettenmoser, and Sheetal Patel. 2017. "Prescription Drug Advertising and Promotion Regulations and Enforcement in Select Global Markets." Food and Drug Law Institute. https://www.fdli.org/2017/08/prescrip tion-drug-advertising-promotion-regulations-enforcement-select-global-markets/.

The authors of this article review statutory requirements for prescription drug advertising in the United States and four other countries: Brazil, Chile, Colombia, and Japan.

"National Prescription Drug Take Back Day." 2020. Diversion Control Division, Drug Enforcement Administration, U.S. Department of Justice. https://www.deadiversion.usdoj.gov/drug_disposal/takeback/.

Each year, the DEA sponsors one or more "take back days," during which the public can return unused drugs at designated areas in their geographical region. This web page provides information on the next upcoming such event, with details on the results of take back days in previous years.

"NIH Policy and Guidelines on the Inclusion of Women and Minorities as Subjects in Clinical Research." 2017. NIH Grants and Funding. https://grants.nih.gov/policy/inclusion/women-and-minorities/guidelines.htm.

This announcement provides details about the history and current status of federal policy on the involvement of women and minorities in clinical drug testing. It is an important resource on this topic on the Internet. For the relevant 1994 document on which this policy is based, see the Federal Register listing at https://www.govinfo.gov/content/pkg/FR-1994-03-09/html/94-5435.htm.

"Orphan Drug Act—Relevant Excerpts." 2018. U.S. Food and Drug Administration. https://www.fda.gov/industry/desig nating-orphan-product-drugs-and-biological-products/orphan-drug-act-relevant-excerpts.

In 1983, the U.S. Congress passed the Orphan Drug Act (21 CFR 316) to provide incentives for drug manufacturers to conduct research for new drugs designed for the treatment of rare diseases and disorders. Today, *rare* means fewer than 1 in 200,000 individuals in the general population.

"Pharmaceutical Fraud." 2020. Whistleblower Law Collective. https://www.whistleblowerllc.com/what-we-do/healthcare-fraud/pharmaceutical-fraud/.

Many opportunities exist for individuals and companies involved in the production, sale, and use of prescription drugs. This website lists some of the most common types of illegal behavior that fall into this category, including illegal off-label use, kickbacks, improper billing, Medicare fraud, and drug rebate fraud.

"Policy of Inclusion of Women in Clinical Trials." 2019. Office on Women's Health. https://www.womenshealth.gov/30-achievements/04.

This short article provides a good overview of the federal policy on the inclusion of women in clinical trials of prescription drugs, with recent changes in those policies.

"Prescription Drug Advertising: Questions and Answers." 2015. U.S. Food and Drug Administration. https://www.fda .gov/drugs/prescription-drug-advertising/prescription-drug-advertising-questions-and-answers.

A Q&A format is used on this website to provide information on questions regarding the regulation by the FDA
of prescription and OTC drug advertising.

"Prescription Drug Pricing." 2020. American Medical
Association. https://www.ama-assn.org/topics/prescription-drug-
pricing.
This website provides access to news items from the
American Medical Association (AMA) with regard to pre-
scription drug pricing. An excellent resource not only for
AMA views on the topic but also for the current status of
the subject overall.

"Prescription Drugs." 2018. Public Health Professionals Gate-
way, Centers for Disease Control and Protection. https://www
.cdc.gov/phlp/publications/topic/prescription.html.
This website focuses on links to a variety of federal and
state prescription drug laws, including doctor shopping
laws, tamper-resistant containers, prescription drug identification laws, pain management clinic regulation, and
prescription drug overdose emergencies.

"Prescription Drugs." 2020. The Commonwealth Fund. https://
www.commonwealthfund.org/prescription-drugs.
The Commonwealth Fund website includes a section
reviewing latest news on a host of topics relating to prescription drugs, such as recent proposed legislation, costs
of prescription drugs, pharmacy policies and practices,
employee benefit plans, and the state of current research
in the field.

"Prescription Drugs." 2020. Gov.track. https://www.govtrack
.us/congress/bills/subjects/prescription_drugs/6184.
The Library of Congress maintains this website, listing
all legislation that has been introduced on a given topic,
in this case, prescription drugs. The list is exhaustive,
consisting of more than one hundred bills introduced in

2019 alone. The predicted prognosis of passage for each bill is also provided, with well over 90 percent of such bills receiving a prognosis of 3 percent or less.

"Prescription Drugs." 2020. U.S. News. https://www.usnews .com/topics/subjects/prescription-drugs.
This website contains links to articles on prescription drugs and related topics that have appeared in recent issues of the *U.S. News and World Report* magazine and website.

"Prescription Drugs: News, Analysis and Opinion from POLITICO." 2020. Politico. https://www.politico.com/news/ prescription-drugs/1.
Politico is a reliable source of information on a variety of topics of everyday interest to consumers. This website contains links to articles from the company dated 2020 on the topic of prescription drugs. The emphasis of those articles is on the political aspects of the subject.

"Prescription Medicines." n.d. National Institute on Drug Abuse. https://www.drugabuse.gov/drug-topics/prescription-medicines.
The National Institute on Drug Abuse is an excellent resource for all aspects of prescription medicines, including information on stimulants, depressants, and opioids; misuse of prescription drugs; the Monitoring the Future study of trends on drug misuse by young adults; drugs facts on opioid drugs, fentanyl, and related topics; medications for the treatment of opioid abuse; and federal funding for research and education on prescription drug abuse.

"Risk Evaluation and Mitigation Strategies: REMS." 2019. U.S. Food and Drug Administration. https://www.fda.gov/ drugs/drug-safety-and-availability/risk-evaluation-and-mit igation-strategies-rems. This website provides a good general introduction to the use of REMS strategies for certain drugs. It includes a link to all drugs currently monitored under the FDA REMS program.

"Safe Supply: Concept Document." 2019. Canadian Association of People Who Use Drugs. https://vancouver.ca/files/cov/capud-safe-supply-concept-document.pdf.

One approach to dealing with the problem of prescription drug abuse is to provide by means of a safe, legal system the drugs to which a person has become addicted. This document provides the theoretical background and basis for that type of program, along with a description of the way in which such a system operates.

Saha, Tiash. 2019. "The Biggest Ever Pharmaceutical Lawsuits." Pharmaceutical Technology. https://www.pharmaceutical-technology.com/features/biggest-pharmaceutical-lawsuits/.

The temptation to cut corners or carry out other activities to increase profits on drug manufacture and sale is always very strong in the prescription drug industry. That fact is illustrated by the number and size of law suits that have been brought by individuals, attorneys, and legal groups against the activities of some prescription drug manufacturers. This website provides an overview of the ten largest penalties issues by courts for some type of illegal pharmaceutical practice. The size of the suits described here ranges from $762 million to $3 billion.

Shepherd, Joanna. 2019. "Pharmacy Benefit Managers, Rebates, and Drug Prices: Conflicts of Interest in the Market for Prescription Drugs." *Yale Law & Policy Review*. 38: 1–28. http://dx.doi.org/10.2139/ssrn.3313828.

The author explores the relationship between pharmacy benefit managers and drug manufacturers that is contributory to the continuing increase in prescription drug prices.

Spiro, Topher, Maura Calsyn, and Thomas Huelskoetter. 2016. "Negotiation Plus: A Framework for Value-Based Drug Pricing Negotiation." Center for American Progress. https://www.americanprogress.org/issues/healthcare/reports/2016/09/26/144760/negotiation-plus-a-framework-for-value-based-drug-pricing-negotiation/.

The Center for American Progress has been concerned about the problem of the increasing costs of prescription drugs for some time. In 2016, it proposed a plan for working with pharmaceutical companies to help solve this problem. That plan, Negotiation Plus, is described and discussed here.

"Statewide Prescription Drug Database: 2015–Present." 2020. National Conference of State Legislatures. https://www.ncsl.org/research/health/prescription-drug-statenet-database.aspx.

The National Conference of State Legislatures provides an ongoing review of the legislation that has been proposed and/or adopted by the nation's fifty state legislatures in thirteen areas: access, biologics and biosimilars; clinical trials and right to try; compounding pharmacy regulation; cost sharing and deductibles—consumers; insurance/coverage—Rx drugs; Medicaid use and cost—Rx drugs; prescription drug measures; pharmacy benefit managers; pricing and payment—industry; safety and errors—Rx drugs; specialty pharmaceuticals; and utilization management—Rx drugs.

"Tag: Prescription Drugs." n.d. Federal Trade Commission. https://www.ftc.gov/industry/prescription-drugs.

Prescription drugs have been and continue to be the topic of many court cases, administrative rulings, public statements, and other documents dealing with their status in U.S. society. This web page provides an up-do-date and complete listing of many (most?) of these documents dating from 2003 to the present day.

Taylor, Paul. 2016. "Do Women Ever Respond Differently than Men to Prescription Drugs?" The Globe and Mail. https://www.theglobeandmail.com/life/health-and-fitness/health-advisor/do-women-ever-respond-differently-than-men-to-prescription-drugs/article32619772/.

> The author answers this question, asked on the newspaper's website. The answer: yes.

"The Truth about Prescription Drug Abuse." 2008. Foundation for a Drug-Free World. http://f.edgesuite.net/data/www.drugfreeworld.org/files/truth-about-prescription-drug-abuse-booklet-en.pdf.

> This booklet is available in hard copy and online. It is designed primarily for young adults and consists mainly of information about specific prescription drugs that are most commonly used illicitly.

Twomey, Madeline. 2019. "Comprehensive Reform to Lower Prescription Drug Prices." Center for American Progress. https://www.americanprogress.org/issues/healthcare/news/2019/01/29/465621/comprehensive-reform-lower-prescription-drug-prices/.

> This article provides a good general introduction to the problem of drug overpricing, along with a review of some programs that have been developed to deal with the problem.

Waldrop, Thomas, and Maura Calsyn. 2020. "State Policy Options to Reduce Prescription Drug Spending." Center for American Progress. https://www.americanprogress.org/issues/healthcare/reports/2020/02/13/480415/state-policy-options-reduce-prescription-drug-spending/.

> Among the variety of efforts being made to reduce the cost of prescription drugs, many programs developed by the states are also important. This article reviews the most common of these efforts.

"Warren, Schakowsky Introduce Bicameral Legislation to Radically Reduce Drug Prices through Public Manufacturing of Prescription Drugs." 2018. Elizabeth Warren. https://www.warren.senate.gov/newsroom/press-releases/warren-schakowsky-introduce-bicameral-legislation-to-radically-reduce-drug-prices-through-public-manufacturing-of-prescription-drugs.

Senator Elizabeth Warren (D-MA) in 2018 introduced a bill in the U.S. Senate for the creation of an independent governmental agency to manufacture prescription drugs, with the ultimate goal of reducing the cost of such products for the American people. This website contains a description of that plan, along with a link to the text of that bill.

"Where and How to Dispose of Unused Medicines." 2020. U.S. Food and Drug Administration. https://www.fda.gov/consumers/consumer-updates/where-and-how-dispose-unused-medicines.

One of the practical everyday issues surrounding the use of prescription drugs is what to do with unused pills and other such medical products. If not properly disposed of, they can be used for illegal recreational purposes, leading to serious medical consequences. This web page provides guidance on to how to deal with unused drugs. A list of locations at which such drugs can be disposed of can be found at https://www.fda.gov/drugs/disposal-unused-medicines-what-you-should-know/drug-disposal-drug-take-back-locations.

Wineinger, Nathan E., Yunyue Zhang, and Eric J. Topol. 2019. "Trends in Prices of Popular Brand-Name Prescription Drugs in the United States." *JAMA Network Open.* 2(5): e194791. doi:10.1001/jamanetworkopen.2019.4791.

This very useful survey reviews trends in the prices of forty-nine of the top-selling prescription drugs in the United States between 2012 and 2017.

Younkin, Peter Allen. 2010. "A Healthy Business: The Evolution of the U.S. Market for Prescription Drugs." [Dissertation]. University of California at Berkeley. https://escholarship.org/uc/item/7zx4c61f.

The author asks how political, social, and technological factors may affect the quantity and types of prescription drugs made available to the U.S. consumer, dating as far back as 1940.

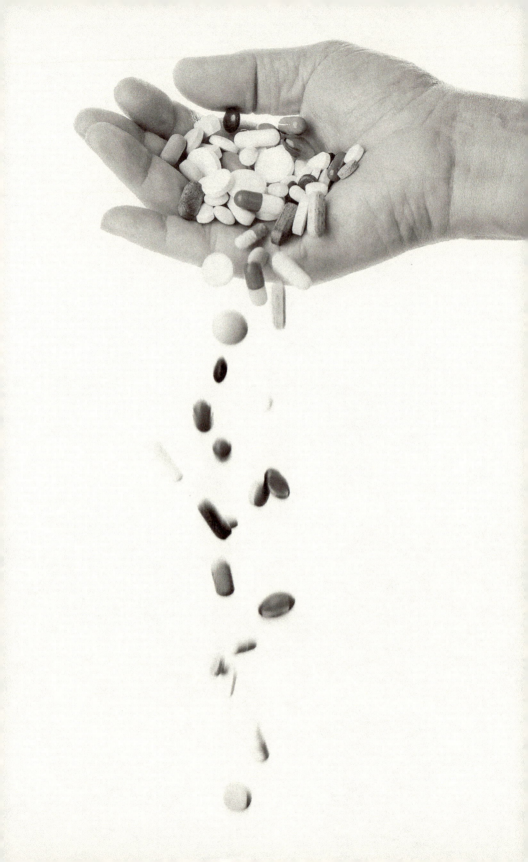

Introduction

The history of written prescriptions and prescription drugs dates at least to the second millennium BCE. This chapter summarizes some of the most important events in that long history.

ca. 2600 BCE   One of the dates suggested for the earliest prescriptions ever written. Clay tablets from the ancient city of Nippur have been found containing several directions for the preparation of medical treatments. Some dispute exists as to whether the artifacts are actually the earliest of tablets of this kind that have been uncovered.

ca. 2000 BCE   A legendary Chinese emperor, Shen Nung, is credited as the author of the first collection of medical prescriptions in Chinese history, the *Shen-nung pen ts'ao ching* ("Divine Husbandman's Materia Medica"). He is said to have developed about 365 preparations consisting of herbs and/or minerals for the treatment of a host of diseases and disorders. Shen is often called the father of Chinese medicine and the father of acupuncture.

ca. 1850 BCE   The Kahun papyrus contains thirty-three prescriptions for the treatment of gynecological disorders dating to the reign of the pharaoh Amenemhet III. The artifact was found at the village of Fayoum in modern-day Egypt.

A very large variety of prescription drugs is now available for the treatment and prevention of disease. (Nikolai Sorokin/Dreamstime.com)

ca. 1550 BCE   The Ebers papyrus, dating to the reign of the pharaoh Amenhotep I (1546–1526 BC), is found in the Valley of the Kings. It contains 877 remedies for a host of diseases and disorder. A sample of the original document and its translation can be found at https://bxscience.edu/ourpages/auto/2008/11/10/43216077/egypt%20medicine.pdf.

ca. 1500 BCE   A statue from the Minoan civilization of the period shows a goddess wearing a crown with three removable capsules that appear to be poppy flowers. The statue's closed eyes suggest to some authorities a state of trance that might be attributed to the use of opium. Substantial evidence exists for the knowledge and use of opium to prehistoric times in Europe and the Middle East.

ca. 600 BCE   The Indian physician Sushruta prepares a medical text now known as *Sushruta Samhita* ("Sushruta's Compendium"), generally regarded as the first medical/herbal text produced in ancient India. His list of prescribed treatments included the use of herbs and minerals, physical procedures, and methods that would now be regarded as "alternative" forms of medicine.

ca. 500 BCE   The first "trademarked" drug is prepared on the Mediterranean island of Lemmos. The substance is made of a type of clay widely used at the time because of its many medical benefits. The clay was so popular, in fact, that it eventually became no longer generally available. When still in use, it was mined, dried, and stamped with a mark of authenticity before being sold to the general public. The product was called *terra sigillata*, or "sealed earth."

50–75 CE   The Roman physician Pedanius Dioscorides compiles one of the first materia medicas ever written and certainly one of the most influential books of this type. In five volumes, the book describes more than six hundred plants and minerals that can be used to produce more than a thousand medicinal substances. His recipes remained in general use until at least the early fifteenth century.

ca. 150 CE   The Greek physician Galen develops techniques for combining and blending a variety of herbs to produce substances for medical use. The procedure is said to be the origin of the process of compounding and is memorialized in the modern use of the term *galenical*, which refers to mixtures of natural substances rather than synthetic materials prepared and used for medical purposes. For more information on the use of galenical medicine in today's world, see https://aromaticstudies.com/galenic-medicine-what-is-it/.

ca. 760 CE   An estimate of when the world's first pharmacy (or drugstore) was founded, in Baghdad. According to one report (https://www.pharmaceutical-journal.com/pharmacy-in-baghdad/20002545.article), the owner and manager of the business was a pharmacist named Isaac Abu Quraysh, private pharmacist to the Abbasid ruler al-Mahdi. Other authorities cite other individuals and dates for this innovation.

1025   The Islamic polymath Abu Ali al-Husayn ibn 'Abd Allah ibn Sina (known in the West as Avicenna) completes his *Canon of Medicine*, a compilation of all medical knowledge available at the time. Avicenna is widely regarded as "the most famous and influential of all the Islamic philosopher-scientists" of all time (https://www.ncbi.nlm.nih.gov/pmc/articles/PMC3952394/). Among his many medical topics is a collection of 650 prescriptions for the treatment of a host of diseases and disorders.

1240   Frederick II of Hohenstaufen, emperor of Germany and king of Sicily, issues a decree separating the professions of pharmacy and medicine, two fields that had previously been practiced by the same individuals.

1345   This date is often mentioned as being the year in which the first apothecary shop in London was formed.

1498   The first official pharmacopoeia, the *Ricettario Fiorentino*, is published in Florence. It is compiled through the joint efforts of the Guild of Physicians and Apothecaries to serve as the official guide for the preparation and use of medications. The work also contains a description of the ideal pharmacist, *D'ingegno et di* *corpo destro, di buoni costumi, non avaro e fedele* ("a person of the correct body, good morals, not stingy and faithful").

1617   King James I of England issues a charter for the formation of a new organization, the Master, Wardens and Society of the Art and Mystery of the Apothecaries of the City of London, the first formal organization of apothecaries in the world. The charter recognizes apothecary practice as a distinct and unique practice from that of medicine, herbalism, and other related occupations of the time.

1653   Dutch surgeon Gysbert van Imbroch begins to offer for sale drugs in his general store in New Amsterdam (now New York City), a step sometimes referred to as the first "drug store" in the United States.

1727   Elizabeth Gooking Greenleaf and her husband open an apothecary shop in Boston, making her the first woman to practice as an apothecary in the United States.

1775   Boston apothecary Andrew Craigie is appointed the first apothecary general for the American army. His job is to collect and manage the army's supply of drugs. The post was abolished in 1821.

1803   German pharmacist Friedrich Sertürner isolates morphine from opium. The experiment is the first such research in which a new type of narcotic alkaloid is extracted from a natural product.

1816   French immigrant Louis Joseph Dufilho Jr. of New Orleans becomes the nation's first licensed pharmacist. He opens his own "drug store" seven years later, sometimes said to be the first such dedicated business in the United States.

1820   A group of physicians meets in Washington, D.C., to construct the United States Pharmacopoeia (USP). The book, *The Pharmacopoeia of the United States of America: 1820*, is designed to provide definitions and standards for medicines commonly in use in the United States. The USP is now used as the standard for drug quality in more than 140 countries around the world.

1821 Sixty-eight Philadelphia pharmacists meet to discuss the creation of an institute for the professional training of members of the profession. Out of that meeting arises the Philadelphia College of Pharmacy, the first institution of its kind in the United States. The college is later renamed and exists today as the University of the Sciences, still located in Philadelphia.

1821 In one of the best known and most important works of its kind, English essayist Thomas De Quincey publishes his *Confessions of an English Opium-Eater*, an autobiographical account of his experiences in the use of opium as a recreational drug.

1848 The U.S. Congress passes the Drug Importation Act. The action was based on reports that large numbers of soldiers died during the Mexican-American War of 1846–1848 because of adulterated drugs that had been shipped to troops from outside the United States were of dubious efficacy and safety.

1849 American pharmacist William Proctor Jr. publishes the first American pharmacology textbook, *Practical Pharmacy*. Because of his widespread influence on the development of the science in the United States, Proctor is sometimes known as the father of American pharmacy.

1852 The American Pharmaceutical Association is founded at the Philadelphia College of Pharmacy. The organization is known today as the American Pharmacists Association.

1890 The Division of Chemistry is created within the U.S. Department of Agriculture. One of the division's primary responsibilities is monitoring the quality and safety of food and drugs. The division is later renamed the Bureau of Chemistry in 1901 and, in 1906, the U.S. Food and Drug Administration (FDA).

1897 German chemist Felix Hoffmann, working at the Bayer company in Germany, for the first time isolates aspirin and heroin within a two-week period. The two compounds—one now an OTC product and the other a prescription drug—soon become the leading products for the company.

1902   The Drug Laboratory is created within the Bureau of Chemistry, part of the U.S. Department of Agriculture. The purpose of the office is to standardize the treatment of drugs and methods for their study within the federal government. The Drug Laboratory is the parent group of what has come to be the Center for Drug Evaluation and Research in the FDA today.

1905   The American Medical Association institutes a voluntary program of drug approval. In order for a product to be advertised in its publications, a pharmaceutical company must submit to the Association documentation that it is both safe and efficacious. The program remained in effect until 1955.

1906   The Pure Food and Drugs Act sets out the first effective regulations for controlling the safety of drugs for sale to the general public. Foods that are misbranded or adulterated are prohibited from interstate commerce.

1911   In *United States v. Johnson* (221 U.S. 488), the U.S. Supreme Court rules that the Pure Food and Drugs Act of 1906 does not prohibit a manufacturer from making false medical claims about a drug; only false statements as to the composition and/or identity of the drug were prohibited.

1912   In response to the Supreme Court ruling about the Pure Food and Drugs Act of 1906 (see **1911**), Congress passes the Sherley Amendment, prohibiting "false and fraudulent" labeling of a product (though not advertising). The Amendment is only partially successful, however, because of the difficulty in proving a supplier's intent for the labeling process.

1914   The Harrison Narcotics Act passes. The Act is one of the most important and best known pieces of legislation relating to the use of drugs in the United States. Its rather modest provisions place limits on the availability of opium and opium products and cocaine as well as has requiring more stringent record keeping by dispensers of such drugs.

1918   New York state passes the first version of a prescription drug monitoring program, in which prescribing physicians were required to use "serially numbered official prescriptions blanks" issued by the state health department to be forwarded by pharmacies to the state for recording. The program remained in effected until 1921.

1937 One hundred seven people die after ingesting a drug known as elixir sulfanilamide. Although widely known as an unsafe concoction, many physicians routinely prescribed the drug. This event was directly related to the passage a year later of a drastic revision of the 1906 Pure Food and Drugs Act.

1938 Largely in response to the elixir sulfanilamide disaster of 1937, the U.S. Congress passes a wide-reaching revision of the 1906 Pure Food and Drugs Act with much greater emphasis on ensuring the safety and efficacy of prescription and other drugs.

1939 California establishes the first continuously operating modern prescription drug monitoring program. A new Bureau of Narcotics Enforcement is created to enforce the program.

1941 Nearly 300 people die from taking the antibiotic sul-fathiazole, which has been contaminated with the sedative phe-nobarbital. The tragedy is instrumental in prompting the FDA to issue a document titled Good Manufacturing Practices. The program remains in existence today, designed to ensure that manufacturers, processors, and packagers of drugs, medical devices, and some food and blood products take steps to ensure that their products are safe, pure, and effective.

1941 The U.S. Congress adopts the so-called Insulin Amendment (613 CFR 506), requiring the testing of insulin products for purity, strength, quality, and identity. The law is one of the earliest pieces of legislation designed to ensure the safety and efficacy of a prescription drug.

1945 The U.S. Congress passes the so-called Penicillin Amendment (59 Stat. 281), extending the program of testing that originated with the Insulin Amendment (see **1941**), to products claimed to consist of or contain penicillin.

1950 In *Alberty Food Products Co. v. U.S.* (194 F.2d 463), the U.S. Court of Appeals for the Ninth Circuit rules that labeling on a drug must indicate the purpose for which the drug is to be used. This decision provides the basis for the modern FDA regulation of "unapproved" and "off-label" drugs as well as health claims for products that have not been approved as drugs.

1951   The U.S. Congress adopts the Durham-Humphrey Amendment, an attempt to clarify the status of prescription drugs in the United States. The Amendment specifies the types of drugs that are to be considered as "prescription" drugs and the mechanisms by which they can be ordered by physicians and sold by pharmacists. The Amendment first clarified the type of drug to which the legislation applied, namely one that is (1) a habit-forming drug, (2) not safe for use except under the supervision of a medical practitioner, or (3) limited to use under the professional supervision of a practitioner licensed by law to administer such drug. The Amendment then specified the conditions under which such drugs could be sold: (1) through a prescription written by a practitioner licensed by law to administer such drug, (2) by means of an oral prescription of such a practitioner, which is reduced promptly to writing and filed by a pharmacist, or (3) by refilling any written or oral prescription that has been authorized by the prescriber.

1954   The FDA creates a voluntary program of adverse drug effects through the efforts of the American Society of Hospital Pharmacists, the American Association of Medical Record Librarians, and the American Medical Association. The program is the first step in the eventual development of post-approval monitoring that now constitutes Stage IV of the FDA drug approval process. By 1963, more than 200 hospitals were voluntarily reporting adverse effects from prescription drug use. The modern manifestation of this program is the Adverse Event Reporting System, fully developed by the FDA in 1998 (qv).

1959   Paul Janssen of the Janssen Pharmaceutica company invents and patents the opioid fentanyl.

1962   The U.S. Congress adopts the Drug Efficacy Amendment to the Federal Food, Drug, and Cosmetics Act of 1938. More commonly known as the Kefauver-Harris Amendment, for its sponsors, the legislation outlines the basics of the drug approval process that remains in effect today.

1966   The Fair Packaging and Labeling Act authorizes the Federal Trade Commission and the FDA to require certain basic information to be included on labeling of all consumer products. The data required include the product contained; the name and place of business of the manufacturer, packer, or distributor; and the net weight or numerical count of contents.

1967   A conference is held in San Francisco titled Ethnopharmacologic Search for Psychoactive Drugs. The meeting focuses on the search for psychoactive compounds in natural substances, such as plants and fungi. The discipline, ethnopharmacology, soon expands to mean the search for any type of healing substance obtained from natural sources, one of the most productive fields of new drug research even today.

1968   In order to comply with the Kefauver-Harris Act of 1962, the FDA begins a study of the efficacy for 4,000 drugs marketed between 1938 and 1962. That ongoing program, the Drug Efficacy Study Implementation (DESI), continues today.

1968   The FDA issues its first "patient package insert" requirement, a requirement that a brief statement of risks and benefits from using the drug be listed. The first drug covered by this regulation was an isoproterenol inhalation device.

1970   In *Upjohn v. Finch*, the drug manufacturer Upjohn argued that one or more of their products should be considered to be "approved" by the FDA because they had been commercially successful, whether or not relevant research data to that effect had been produced and/or filed. The U.S. Supreme Court differed with that view and said that "commercial success" in and of itself was not sufficient to prove the safety and efficacy of a drug.

1972   The FDC begins the Over the Counter Drug Review, a program similar to DESI (**1968**), focusing on over-the-counter products rather than on prescription drugs.

1977   The FDA issues guidelines banning the participation of women of childbearing age from clinical research studies. The purpose of the rule was to protect such individuals from possible deleterious effects of new drug products. The policy was revised and largely rescinded in 1991.

1981   The FDA promulgates the Common Rule. The rule is a statement of the ethical issues to be considered in the use of humans in biomedical and behavioral research. It appears in its final form in Title 45 CFR 46 (Public Welfare), Subparts A, B, C, and D, issued in 1991. It is now a required component of all federally funded research as well as research programs in most private and independent colleges, universities, corporations, and other funding agencies.

1983   The U.S. Congress passes the Orphan Drug Act. The Act provides incentives for drug companies to conduct research on and to produce drugs for diseases and disorders that occur relatively infrequently in the general population. The FDA currently defines "infrequently" as fewer than 1 case per 200,000 persons in the general population. Among the tax incentives are extension of patent rights for a drug, tax incentives, and waivers on drug approval fees.

1984   The Drug Price Competition and Patent Term Restoration Act (also known as the Hatch-Waxman Act) allows the FDA to approve generic versions of brand-name drugs without repeating the research that proved the safety and effectiveness of the original brand-name drugs. This provision improves the willingness of drug manufacturers to invest in the production of less expensive (and, therefore, less profitable) generic equivalents of brand-name drugs. The Act also created benefits to brand-name companies, by allowing them to apply for up to five years' additional patent protection for the new medicines they developed to make up for time lost while their products were going through FDA's approval process.

1987 The FDA issues regulations for the process to be followed in the submission of a new candidate drug for its approval. The regulations outline the basic procedure by which drugs are approved by the FDA today. The document described in the regulation is the Investigational New Drug (IND) application. It defines and explains the phases (clinical trials) through which a candidate molecule must pass before being assessed by the FDA.

1987 The Center for Drug Evaluation and Research is created with the Food and Drug Administration. The Center is the agency through which applications for new drugs pass and are approved or rejected.

1987 The FDA revises its regulations with respect to IND applications. It outlines provisions for providing experimental drugs to patients with serious diseases for whom no alternative therapies are currently available. The program is currently described as the FDA's Expanded Access Program for Investigational Drugs. The original legislation can be found at 21 CFR 312, 314, 511, and 514.

1988 The Prescription Drug Marketing Act bans the diversion of prescription drugs from legitimate commercial channels. Such actions in the past have been responsible for the sale of mislabeled, adulterated, subpotent, and counterfeit drugs to the public. Among the provisions of the new law are a requirement that drug wholesalers be licensed by the states; restriction of reimportation from other countries to the United States; and bans on the sale, trade, or purchase of drug samples and traffic or counterfeiting of redeemable drug coupons.

1991 The FDA issues new guidelines for the participation of women of childbearing age in clinical research studies (see **1977**).

1992 The Congress adopts the Prescription Drug User Fee Act. The Act sets fees to be paid by drug companies for the approval process through which candidate molecules pass in the FDA. The Act must be renewed every five years, and during that process, user fees may be adjusted as needed by the

FDA. In 2021, user fees for drugs for which clinical data were required were $2,875,842, with an addition program fee of $336,432.

1993   The FDA issues guidelines suggesting that clinical trials for new drugs include sufficient numbers of males and females to detect any possible differences in drug effects based on sex. In addition, the guidelines recommend that sex differences detected during trials be reported to the federal government.

1997   The Food and Drug Administration Modernization Act consists of a number of provisions to make the FDA better able to deal with prescription drug–related problems in the twenty-first century. It includes legislation on prescription drug user fees, off-label use, pharmacy compounding, food safety and labeling, and standards for medical products.

1998   The FDA implements the Adverse Event Reporting System (AERS), a computerized system by which health care professionals, consumers, and other interested parties can report adverse events apparently resulting from the use of some approved FDA product. The system allows the FDA to monitor possible long-term or otherwise unexpected harmful results of the use of an approved product.

1998   The FDA issues the Demographic Rule, a monitoring system designed to ensure that individuals of all age, gender, and race are fairly represented in clinical trials of new drugs. Data to be reported cover the safety and efficacy of such drugs for all groups.

1998   The FDA issues the Pediatric Rule. The rule was designed to ensure that drugs presented for approval to the FDA be both safe and efficacious for children as well as adults. The Rule was invalidated four years later by a court that found the FDA to have overstepped the bounds of its authority. Further attempts to achieve the objectives of this Rule were proposed over the next five years, resulting eventually in the passage of the Pediatric Research Equity Act of 2003.

1999   As one provision of the Food and Drug Administration Modernization Act of 1997, the website ClinicalTrials.gov is created to provide information about the existence and operation of clinical drug trials, along with instructions for applying to participate in such trials.

2000   As a way of protecting American consumers from tainted or otherwise unsafe imported drugs, the U.S. Congress passes the Medicine Equity and Drug Safety Act. The Act prohibits the import of any drugs from foreign countries to the United States except for shipments from American companies that originally produced the drug.

2002   As a way of encouraging the development of safe and efficacious drugs for children (also see **1998**, the Pediatric Rule), Congress adopts the Best Pharmaceuticals for Children Act. The Act allows the FDA to grant an innovative drug company an additional six months of patent exclusiveness for drugs that have been tested especially with children.

2003   The U.S. Congress adopts the Pediatric Research Equity Act (PREA), one of many attempts to write a court-approved approach to the development of safe and efficacious drugs for children. The Act allows the FDA to require additional testing on children of new drug candidates if there is evidence that the drug is likely to be used by a "substantial number" of children. The value for that "substantial number" is eventually set at 50,000.

2003   The Medicare Prescription Drug, Improvement, and Modernization Act (also known simply as Medicare Modernization Act of 2003), creates Medicare Part D, a system for providing drug benefits to Medicare participants. It also specifically prohibits federal officials from negotiating drug prices with pharmaceutical companies.

2004   The Project BioShield Act authorizes the FDA to expedite its review procedures to enable rapid distribution of drugs needed for countermeasures to chemical, biological, and nuclear agents that may be used in a terrorist attack against the United States.

2005   The Drug Safety Board is created to advise the director of the Center for Drug Evaluation and Research on issues relating to drug safety and for the distribution of information on drug safety to health professionals and patients.

2006   The first biosimilar medicine, Omnitrope, is approved for use. Biosimilars, also known as biologics, are drugs that are similar to other biological medicines that have already been authorized for use by some authorizing agency, such as the FDA.

2006   The Institute for Clinical and Economic Review (ICER) is founded for the purpose of studying, monitoring, and making recommendations on prescription drugs, medical tests, and other health care delivery innovations.

2010   In response to the continued spread of drug abuse in the United States, President Barack Obama announces the creation of a National Drug Control Policy. In addition to reiterating and strengthening drug enforcement policies and practices, the program is designed to place greater emphasis on "aggressive prevention and recovery programs."

2010   The state of Florida passes the nation's first pill mill law.

2010   A second "wave" of the opioid epidemic begins in the United States. The wave is characterized by a use predominantly of heroin by drug abusers.

2012   The Food and Drug Administration Safety and Innovation Act authorizes the FDA to collect user fees from the medical industry to fund reviews of innovator drugs, medical devices, generic drugs, and biosimilar biologics. It also establishes a system for the expedited review of innovative drugs designed for certain rare pediatric diseases.

2012   Kentucky becomes the first state to pass a so-called doctor shopping law.

2013   A third "wave" of the opioid epidemic begins in the United States. The wave is characterized by a use predominantly of fentanyl by drug abusers.

2013   In response to a 2012 outbreak of fungal meningitis, the U.S. Congress passes the Drug Quality and Security Act. The Act creates a national interactive system for the distribution and sharing of information about drug safety in the United States.

2013   A long-term study by the FDA on inequities in sex and racial representations found no significant disparities for the former category but continuing inequities for race and ethnic groups.

2016   A consortium of more than two dozen federal agencies and private associations joined to form the Diverse Women in Clinical Trials Initiative, an organization designed to encourage more women to volunteer for prescription drug trials.

2018   The Committee on Ensuring Patient Access to Affordable Drug Therapies of the National Academies of Sciences, Engineering, and Medicine publishes a major report *Making Medicines Affordable: A National Imperative*, which reviews the problem of growing prescription drug costs and possible solutions for that problem.

2019   President Donald Trump signs a set of four Executive Orders designed to help bring under control the rising cost of prescription drugs. They dealt with (1) the importance of drugs to the United States, (2) the pricing of insulin and injectable epinephrine, (3) rebates on certain drugs for Medicare Part D beneficiaries, and (4) index-pricing for physician-administered drugs under Plan B of Medicare.

2019   The U.S. House of Representatives passes the Elijah E. Cummings Lower Drug Costs Now Act by a vote of 230 to 192. The Senate declines to consider the bill, meaning that it has died in this session of the Congress.

2020   Governor Gavin Newsom (D-CA) proposes the creation of a state-owned and -operated drug label company as a way of dealing with rising drug costs in the state (and country). The state legislature later adopts legislation requiring the state's Health and Human Services Agency to develop plans for working with drug suppliers and distributors to find ways of increasing competition, lowering prices, and reducing shortages of generic drugs but not to establish a state drug label.

Books, articles, web pages, and other resources on prescription drugs often use terminology that is unfamiliar or that has somewhat different meanings than those of everyday life. This chapter presents several terms used in discussions of prescription drugs, most of which appear in this book. Other terms are also listed for the benefit of readers who continue their research on this topic in other resources.

active ingredient   The component of a drug that produces some biological, chemical, or other effect on the body.

addiction   A long-lasting and typically recurring psychological and/or physiological need for one or more substances, such as alcohol, tobacco, or opioids, that generally results in permanent or long-lasting changes in the neurochemistry of the brain.

adulteration   The process of substituting a substance in whole or in part with another substance with little or no effect expected from the drug and, in some cases, with additional risk to the user.

alternative payment model (APM)   A system for determining the price of a product, such as a prescription drug, that differs from the more traditional approach of allowing the manufacturer of the product to determine the price strictly on their own criterion or criteria.

analgesic   A drug that relieves pain.

analog   In the field of biochemistry, a substance with a chemical structure similar to that of some other substance but with different properties.

annual limit   The maximum amount of money an insurer will pay toward a person's drug expenses in one calendar year.

apothecary   An individual who prepares and sells drugs for medicinal purposes. The term is also used to describe the physical setting in which such a person works. An apothecary differs from a pharmacist in that an apothecary actually makes the drugs to be dispensed, in contrast to simply filling an order issued by a health care specialist. Synonyms for *apothecary* as a site of business include *drug store* and *chemist shop* (especially in Great Britain).

approval letter   The communication sent by the FDA to a drug manufacturer that allows marketing of a new product.

benefits   The types of services an insurer will cover under some given health insurance policy.

Big Pharma   *See* **pharma**.

biological product   *See* **biologics**.

biologics   Drugs that are obtained from humans or other animals, microorganisms, or other living organisms. Some examples include proteins, blood, blood components, genes, and tissues. Also known as a **biologic product**.

biosimilar   A drug or other product that can be shown to be similar to or interchangeable with a product already approved by the FDA. The approval process for biosimilars is substantially easier and faster than that for a completely new drug.

black box warning   Statements found on the insert that comes with a medication, surrounded by a black border and printed in bold type. The statement warns of possible serious safety risk involved in use of the drug and special precautions to be followed in its use.

brand-name drug   A prescription or an over-the-counter (OTC) drug sold by a company with a specific name and/or trademark. Also known as a *proprietary drug*.

candidate molecule   A molecule that is derived from a list of lead candidates as a promising material for additional pharmacological, toxicological, and otherwise clinical testing in the process of drug development. Also, **preclinical candidate**.

catastrophic coverage   A form of health insurance designed to pay for abnormally large medical costs, such a major surgeries or long-term health care for chronic diseases.

causative agent   An organism or chemical that is responsible for the onset of some disease.

chemist   Synonym for *pharmacist*, especially in Great Britain.

coinsurance   The portion of a medical bill that an insured person must pay for some service, above and beyond costs paid by an insurer.

compounding   The process of combining, mixing, or altering ingredients to create a medication tailored to the needs of an individual patient. Compounding includes the combining of two or more drugs.

contraindication   Any condition or circumstance that makes it inadvisable to recommend, prescribe, or use some specific medication. *Also see* **indication**.

deductible   The amount a person has to pay on her or his medical bills for a year before the insurance company begins paying their share of those expenses.

delayed release technology   *See* **modified release technology**.

dependence   A condition in which an individual develops a fixation on or craving for a drug that is not necessarily so severe as to be classified as an addiction but that may, nonetheless, require professional help to overcome.

designer drugs   Illicitly produced drugs with chemical structures similar to those of existing psychoactive substances and pharmacological effects similar to those of such drugs. Also known as **new psychoactive substances**.

donut hole   The period of time during which an insured person is responsible for paying some higher portion of the cost of prescription drugs until the insured has spent enough to qualify for catastrophic coverage (q.v.).

dosage   The size and/or frequency with which a medication should be taken by a user.

drug   A chemical substance used to create some biological effect on an organism. That effect may be either positive (cure or mitigation of a condition) or negative (disabling or addiction). *Also see* **medication**.

drug supply chain   The collection of events through which a prescription drug is supplied to a consumer from a drug manufacturer.

elixir   In general, any solution intended to cure some ailment. The term is most commonly associated with substances thought to have magical effects on a person's health. No longer used in the pharmaceutical industry.

financial toxicity   A term used to describe problems that a person may have because of the cost of medical care. One example is the possibility of large debt and bankruptcy for individuals who are unable to pay the costs of their medical care.

formulary   An official list of drugs approved for general use. Today, the term refers most specifically to the list of prescription drugs covered by some health insurance plan. That list changes on a regular basis, from year to year.

generic company   A drug manufacturer whose primary activity is to produce and sell generic drugs similar to prescription drugs that have been approved by the FDA.

generic drug   A prescription drug that is chemically equivalent to a brand-name drug and has the same dosage, safety, strength, route of administration, quality, performance characteristics, and intended use as the brand-name drug.

half life   The period of time over which the concentration or amount of a drug in the body is reduced to one-half of a given concentration or amount.

Health plant Any formal system for the delivery of health care to individuals, such as Medicare or medigap plans.

Iatrogenic addiction Addiction that occurs as the result of some medical treatment, with or without a health care giver's intent.

Indication Any condition or circumstance that makes it advisable to recommend, prescribe, or use some medication.

Innovator company A drug manufacturer whose primary goal is to invent new prescription drugs, in contrast to the type of work performed by a **generic company** (q.v.).

labeling (drug) Any or all written, printed, or graphic materials found on a drug container or wrapper. It includes contents, indications, effects, dosages, routes, methods, frequency and duration of administration, warnings, hazards, contraindications, side effects, precautions, and other relevant information.

Medicaid Drug Rebate Program A program by which drug manufacturers sign an agreement with the federal government that they will provide a rebate to states in exchange for the federal government's listing the drug as an approved drug under the Medicaid program.

Medicare prescription drug benefit *See* **Part D.**

medication A chemical substance used to prevent, alleviate, or cure some medical condition. Medications differ from drugs in that the former have only positive effects, while the latter may have either positive or negative effects. *Also see* **drug.**

modified release technology A method of making drugs in such a way that the active ingredient in the product is released slowly over a period of time, making possible continuous action of the drug without further ingestion of the substance. Also known as **delayed release technology.**

monograph Defined by the FDA as "drugs that are safe and effective for use by the general public without seeking treatment by a health professional." They are roughly comparable to labeling required of prescription drugs.

narcotic Any drug that affects a person's mood or behavior. Today, the term has been equated with a specific family of drugs with that effect: the opioids.

neurochemistry The study of changes that take place in the structure and function of the brain's nervous system.

neuron A nerve cell.

neurotransmitter A chemical that carries a nerve impulse between two neurons.

new psychoactive substances *See* **designer drugs**.

nonmedical use The taking of a prescription drug, whether obtained by prescription or otherwise, (1) other than in the manner in which it was intended to be taken, (2) other than for the reasons or time period prescribed, (3) or by a person for whom the drug was not prescribed.

off-label drug use Use of a medication in a manner not specifically approved by the FDA as indicated on its packaging label or insert.

online pharmacy A drug delivery system that operates over the Internet, providing prescriptions and orders of drugs to customers through shipping companies and by mail. An online pharmacy may or may not be operating legally.

opiate Any drug obtained from or related to opium.

opioid A synthetic narcotic with chemical, biological, and other properties similar to that of opium but not derived from that compound.

out-of-pocket costs The portion of a medical charge to be paid by an insured person, above and beyond any costs paid by the insurer. *Also see* **coinsurance**.

pain management A term used to describe all methods and materials used to reduce or control the severity of pain suffered by an individual. Prescription drugs are a crucial element in that system.

Part D   A section of the U.S. government's Medicare program designed to help qualified individuals pay for self-administered prescription drugs through prescription drug insurance premiums. Also called the Medicare prescription drug benefit.

patent medicine   A nonprescription drug that is protected by a trademark, usually without precise detailed data about its ingredients and little or no guarantee of efficacy. Sometimes known as a *nostrum*.

pharma   (or **Pharma**) A term used to describe the pharmaceutical industry in toto. Sometimes used in a pejorative sense for the industry. Also called **Big Pharma**.

pharmaceutical equivalents   Two or more forms of a drug that (1) contain the same active ingredient(s), (2) are of the same dosage form and route of administration, and (3) are identical in strength or concentration.

pharmacist   An individual who dispenses prescription and OTC drugs ordered by some other medical specialist. *Also see* **apothecary**.

pharmacology   The study of the characteristics, sources, mode of action, and other properties of drugs.

pharmacopoeia   A book, most commonly published by or under authority of some governmental agency, with information about drugs and other materials used in medicine. This information may include chemical formulas, directions for production, tests for strength and purity, and uses.

pharmacovigilance   All practices associated with determining, monitoring, and controlling the possible adverse effects associated with use of a drug.

pharmacy benefit manager   An organization that is responsible for administering prescription drug programs for commercial health plans, self-insured employer drug plants, Medicare Part D plans, and similar programs. The organization has a multitude of responsibilities, ranging from the creation of formularies to negotiating discounts and rebates with drug manufacturers.

preclinical candidate   *See* **candidate molecule**.

prescription   Written instructions from a physician, dentist, or other qualified health care worker to a pharmacist stating the name, form, dosage strength, and other features of a drug to be issued to a specific patient.

prescription abbreviation   A set of letters and/or numbers used by a prescriber and pharmacist to indicate the correct use of a drug. Some examples include the following: ac ("before meals"), bid or BID ("twice a day), DR ("delayed release"), guttat. ("drop-by-drop"), and qid or QID ("four times a day").

prior authorization   Approval issued by a health insurance company that it will pay for the purchase of drugs prescribed by a health care provider.

proprietary drug   *See* **brand-name drug**.

psychoactive   Having the ability to affect one's mood, behavior, or other mental process.

retail prescription drugs   Prescription drugs that are provided by independent pharmacies, chain pharmacies, food stores, and mass merchandisers. The term does not include prescriptions dispensed in clinics, hospitals, physicians' offices, or pharmacies within a closed health care system.

risk management and mitigation   Any system for identifying the risk posed by a prescription or an OTC drug, including notations on a drug label of potential benefits and risks of the drug. The system includes suggested methods for reducing the type and amount of risk posed by any particular drug or procedure.

semi-synthetic drug   A type of medication produced by making some type of modification in a naturally occurring product in order to change its physical, chemical, biological, or other properties.

snake oil   A substance, often sold by traveling salesmen, with a host of purported benefits for human health but with little or no actual effects on the human body. The term has come to mean any product offered for sale with the primary benefit of making a profit for the salesperson and with little or no benefit to the purchaser.

synergy   An interaction between two or more drugs such that the overall effect of the drugs is greater than the simple sum of those effects. Synergistic effects may be either positive or negative.

synthetic drug   A type of medication made entirely in the laboratory, using no natural product as a raw material in the process.

therapeutic   Relating to any substance or treatment that is likely to have some positive effect on a person's health.

tincture   A medicinal substance consisting of some therapeutic substance dissolved in alcohol.

tolerance   A condition that occurs as the result of continued use of a drug such that (1) increased amounts of the substance are needed in order to achieve some desired effect or (2) a markedly diminished effect occurs with continued use of the same amount of the substance.

toxicity   The degree to which some given substance can cause harm to the human body.

user fee (FDA)   A fee originally (1992) authorizing the U.S. Food and Drug Administration to charge fees to drug manufacturers to expedite the review and approval of new prescription drug applications. The scope of such fees have since been expanded to include a range of human and animal products, including brand-name drugs, biosimilars, generic drugs, and veterinary products.

vaccine   A substance used to stimulate the body's immune system as a way of preventing some disease.

value-based pricing   A method for determining the asking price of a product, such as a prescription drug, based on its perceived benefit to a consumer rather than based on some other criterion, such as profit to the maker of the product.

withdrawal   In the parlance of drugs, a set of symptoms that develop when a person stops using a drug or drugs to which the person has become addicted or on which the person has grown dependent. Symptoms differ depending on individual characteristics of the person involved.

About the Author

David E. Newton holds an associate's degree in science from Grand Rapids (Michigan) Junior College, a B.A. in chemistry (with high distinction), an M.A. in education from the University of Michigan, and an Ed.D. in science education from Harvard University. He is the author of more than 400 textbooks, encyclopedias, resource books, research manuals, laboratory manuals, trade books, and other educational materials.

He taught mathematics, chemistry, and physical science in Grand Rapids, Michigan, for 13 years; was professor of chemistry and physics at Salem State College in Massachusetts for 15 years; and was adjunct professor in the College of Professional Studies at the University of San Francisco for 10 years.

Some of the author's previous books for ABC-CLIO include *Eating Disorders in America* (2019), *Natural Disasters* (2019), *Vegetarianism and Veganism* (2019), *Gender Inequality* (2019), *Birth Control* (2019), *The Climate Change Debate* (2020), *World Oceans* (2020), *GMO Food* (2021), and *Hate Groups* (2021). His other books include *Physics: Oryx Frontiers of Science Series* (2000), *Sick!* (4 vols., 2000), *Science, Technology, and Society: The Impact of Science in the 19th Century* (2 vols., 2001), *Encyclopedia of Fire* (2002), *Molecular Nanotechnology: Oryx Frontiers of Science Series* (2002), *Encyclopedia of Water* (2003), *Encyclopedia of Air* (2004), *The New Chemistry* (6 vols., 2007), *Nuclear Power* (2005), *Stem Cell Research* (2006), *Latinos in the Sciences, Math, and Professions* (2007), and *DNA Evidence and Forensic Science* (2008). He has also been an updating and consulting editor on a number of books and reference works, including *Chemical Compounds* (2005), *Chemical Elements* (2006), *Encyclopedia of Endangered Species* (2006), *World of Mathematics* (2006), *World of Chemistry* (2006), *World of Health* (2006), *UXL Encyclopedia of Science* (2007), *Alternative Medicine* (2008), *Grzimek's Animal Life Encyclopedia* (2009), *Community Health* (2009), *Genetic Medicine* (2009), *The Gale Encyclopedia of Medicine* (2010–2011), *The Gale Encyclopedia of Alternative Medicine* (2013), *Discoveries in Modern Science: Exploration, Invention, and Technology* (2013–2014), and *Science in Context* (2013–2014).